Skin Care

Francine Brown

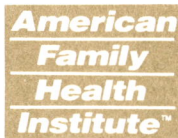

Medical Board

Stanley J. Dudrick, MD
Clinical Professor of Surgery
University of Texas Medical School, Houston, Texas

Jo Eland, RN, PhD
Assistant Professor, University of Iowa
Iowa City, Iowa

Dennis E. Leavelle, MD
Consulting Pathologist, Department of Laboratory Medicine
Mayo Clinic, Rochester, Minnesota

Julena Lind, MN, RN
Director of Education, Center for Health Information, Education and Research
at California Medical Center, Los Angeles, California

Ara G. Paul, PhD
Dean, College of Pharmacy, University of Michigan
Ann Arbor, Michigan

Richard Payne, MD
Clinical Assistant Neurologist, Memorial Sloan-Kettering Cancer Center
New York, New York

William R. Truscott, MD
Diplomate, American Academy of Family Practice, Lansdale Medical Group
Lansdale, Pennsylvania

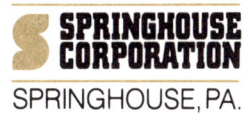

SPRINGHOUSE, PA.

Program Director
Stanley Loeb

Clinical Director
Barbara McVan, RN

Art Director
John Hubbard

Editorial Services Supervisor
David Moreau

Production Manager
Wilbur Davidson

Editors
Jay Hyams
Susan Cass

The charter of the American Family Health Institute is to research and produce high-quality publications that enhance the health of individuals and their families. Essential to health are physical, emotional, and social well-being, not just the absence of illness or infirmity. The Institute's Medical Board has produced the *Health and Fitness* books to share up-to-date and authoritative information that can give readers greater personal control over their health maintenance.

© 1986 by Springhouse Corporation, 1111 Bethlehem Pike, Springhouse, Pa. 19477

All rights reserved. Reproduction in whole or part by any means whatsoever without written permission of the publisher is prohibited by law. Printed in the United States of America.

Library of Congress Cataloging-in-Publication Data
Brown, Francine, 1927-
   Skin care.
    (Health and fitness series)
    Includes index.
    1. Skin—Care and hygiene.   2. Skin—Diseases—Popular works. I. Brunner, Lillian Sholtis.   II. American Family Health Institute. Medical Board. III. Title. IV. Series.
[DNLM: 1. Dermatology—popular works. WR 100 B877s]
RL87.B73   1986   616.5   85-30266
ISBN 0-87434-021-7

The procedures and explanations given in this publication are based on research and consultation with medical and nursing authorities. To the best of our knowledge, these procedures and explanations reflect currently accepted medical practice; nevertheless, they can't be considered absolute and universal recommendations. For individual application, treatment suggestions must be considered in light of the individual's health, subject to a doctor's specific recommendations. The authors and the publisher disclaim responsibility for any adverse effects resulting directly or indirectly from the suggested procedures, from any undetected errors, or from the reader's misunderstanding of the text.

Contents

Skin Care

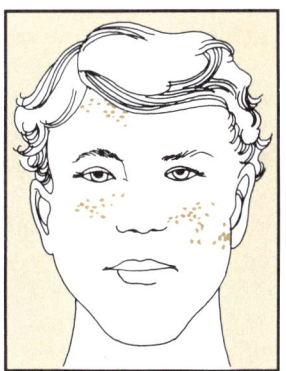

1. What skin is and what it does 4
2. Caring for your skin 11
3. Skin emergencies 25
4. Acne 32
5. Sunburn and sun poisoning 36
6. Allergy-related disorders 41
7. Virus-related disorders 52
8. Common skin problems 62
9. Serious disorders 83

Index 94

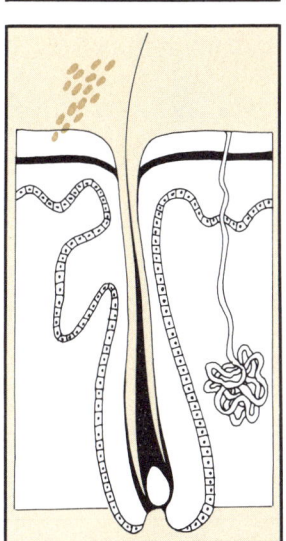

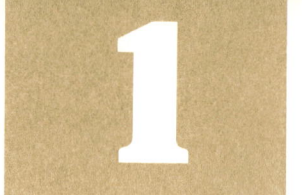

What skin is and what it does

What exactly is your skin? It's the largest, heaviest organ of your body and one of the most efficient and complex. A living, functioning organism, skin is intimately related to all your other bodily organs. Additionally, skin is the covering of your body and the house you live in all your life.

Along the way, it may look smooth and glowing, wrinkled and worn, bumpy or discolored. It may, at times, be in need of treatment or repairs. Much of the time, our skin problems are our own doing.

Any day, we might subject our skin to mistreatment. We might expose it to extreme temperatures, scrape it, scrub it, pinch it, pull it, bend it, scorch it—and then we're surprised and annoyed when it rebels. In fact, when that happens, we tend to ignore its symptoms or trouble.

How big is your skin?
Your skin weighs almost twice as much as either your brain or your liver. If spread out flat, the skin's total area for an average adult would measure approximately 21 square feet and weigh approximately 9 pounds.

Your skin's jobs
Your skin has many jobs to perform, from protecting you to nourishing you. Because of its variety of jobs, your skin has a mix of qualities, depending on the part of your body you examine. Here, your skin is soft, smooth, fragile. There, it's tough and strong.

Your skin is connected to your nervous and circulatory systems and sends your brain reliable reports on your physical, mental, and emotional states. Consider, for example, how you may turn pale with fear, flush with anger, blush with embarrassment, sweat with anxiety.

Then, too, your skin can tell a doctor about a vast array of internal illnesses. Respiratory, cardiac, circulatory, allergic, digestive, glandular, malignant, venereal, and mental disorders are but a part of the list.

In one square inch of skin

If you're interested in lists of facts, you'll want to know that each square inch of human skin contains:
19,500,000 cells
19,500 sensory cells at the ends of nerve fibers
2,000 oil glands
1,300 nerve endings to register pain
650 sweat glands
165 pressure sensors
100 sebaceous glands (to supply the lubricant sebum)
78 nerves
78 sensors for heat
65 hairs and muscles
20 blood vessels, adding up to 15 feet
13 sensors for cold

The skin's layers

The outer layer of the epidermis is made up of dead cells that flake away all the time. Beneath the flaking layer, the epidermis's living cells grow outward and gradually form the layer of dead skin called the keratin.

Underneath is the dermis, which consists of a network of collagen tissue fibers with interweaving blood and lymph vessels, sweat and sebaceous glands, and hair follicles and nerve endings.

Below the dermis is a layer of fat-storage cells called the subcutaneous tissue.

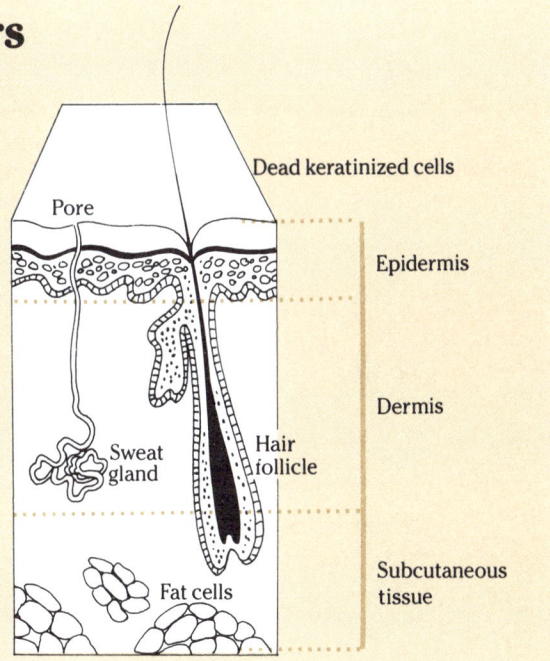

How a hair stands on end

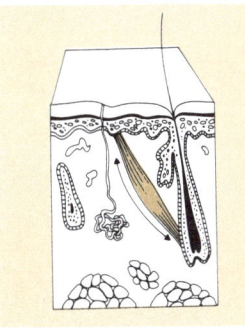

The hair follicle in the dermis is a tube with a central core of dead, keratinized cells that are pushed upward as new cells are produced to form a hair. Each follicle has a small muscle that can contract to make the hair stand upright. Only the palms of the hands and soles of the feet have no hair.

The skin's layers

The outer layers of the skin are called the epidermis, or cuticle. This is the visible part, tough and resilient. However, the degree of toughness varies from one area of the body to another. The scalp, soles of the feet, and palms of the hands are thickest, and the skin of the eyelids is thinnest.

Underneath the epidermis is the dermis, or corium, and below that is a third layer called the subcutaneous tissue. The skin performs most of its work in these lower layers. Fibrous elastic tissue, sometimes containing muscles, can cause your hairs to stand on end. Here, too, are follicles containing hair roots and the pigments that give you your complexion shade. In these lower layers are blood vessels; lymph glands; fat; sweat glands; oil glands that produce sebum, a lubricating secretion; and the nerve endings that provide you with the sensations of touch, pain, heat, and cold.

Each of these skin layers is subdivided into additional layers. One of these layers within a layer, called the basal cell layer, contains most of the skin pigment, or melanin. Melanin determines the degree of color, or pigmentation, in your skin. You can think of melanin as the key to how your skin tans in the sun.

What does your skin do for you?

Your skin works constantly and efficiently at a number of essential activities, such as:

• Regulating body temperature

Your body generates heat through its performance. Your digestive processes, for example, generate as much as 2,500 units of heat, called calories, every day. This heat must be released from your body to maintain an even body temperature around 98.6 degrees F. When the air around you is warm, your body rids itself of excess heat. Nerve endings in your skin alert your nervous system, and your blood vessels enlarge, releasing heat. This process causes flushing or redness of the skin. When the air is cool, your body saves heat by constricting your blood vessels.

• Protecting your inner organs, bones, muscles, and blood vessels

Our daily lives subject us to a variety of bumps and knocks that, without our protective covering, could injure the vital parts within. The skin, because of its thickness and flexibility, is capable of absorbing most of the shock of a direct blow.

• Preventing germs and toxic substances from penetrating to deeper tissues while preventing body fluids from escaping

Your skin forms a barrier that keeps out some harmful organisms and material. Your skin plays an opposite role, too, keeping necessary body fluids, such as blood and water, from leaking, oozing, or gushing out of your body.

• Absorbing small amounts of applied medications

Although the skin keeps out certain injurious elements, it allows many substances in, such as topical medications.

• Helping your body's immune system

Your skin is part of your body's immune defense system. It functions so that foreign protein substances entering it—such as insect venom—are destroyed by the antigen response.

• Producing Vitamin D from the sun's rays

Your skin supplies much of your body's Vitamin D requirements by producing a substance that changes to

Protection from bumps
The skin of your scalp is some of your body's thickest and toughest skin. It serves an important purpose, of course—protecting your head from hard knocks and bumps.

Pathways of pain

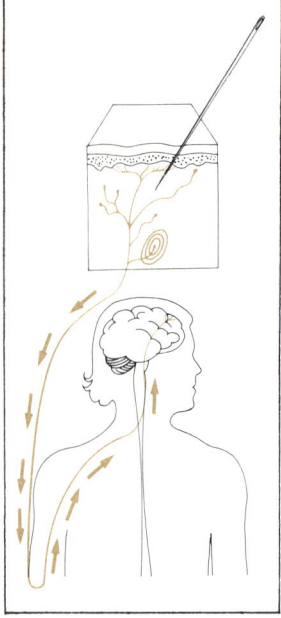

When the nerves in the skin sense injury, a message is sent along the complex system of nerves to the brain. The brain receives this message as pain and sends a message back to the finger to stop the pain. Because of the sensory information your skin gives you, you'll withdraw your hand from something harmful before severe damage is done.

Topical medications are medications applied directly to the skin.

An *antigen* is a substance that stimulates the body's production of antibodies, which combat invading substances.

Vitamin D when exposed to the ultraviolet radiation in sunlight.

• Eliminating body wastes through more than 2 million pores

The skin excretes organic salts, acids, and certain other minerals through perspiration. Depending on the warmth or cold of the weather, an adult produces between 1 and 2 quarts of sweat each day. Also, the amount of physical exercise and degree of emotional stress affect sweat production.

• Providing you with sensory information

You have your own marvelous computer utilizing "software" such as nerve endings, nerves, pressure sensors, sensory cells, and sensors for heat and cold. Your skin provides constant input: "It's hot." "It's cold." "It's soft." "It's smooth." If you were blindfolded and wore earplugs, your skin would allow you to identify objects (needle, pillow, ice cube) and warn you of danger and give sensations of pleasure. Numerous nerve endings under the skin send messages to your brain. As a result, your muscles can react with a prompt and appropriate response.

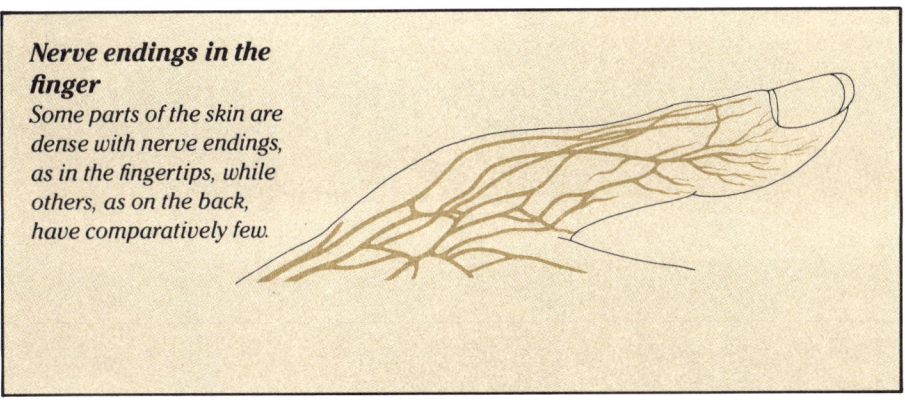

Nerve endings in the finger
Some parts of the skin are dense with nerve endings, as in the fingertips, while others, as on the back, have comparatively few.

• Absorbing the sun's rays and converting them into more melanin (dark pigment)

This tanning process provides a toughened, rougher skin layer that will protect you from future burning.

• Protecting itself from wear and tear

The skin can thicken its own layers in response to wear and tear on the body. (The thick skin on the soles of your feet and hands is an example of skin thickened to provide protection.) Blisters are protective fluid-filled "cushions" produced by the skin to protect itself from burn and pressure damage. The calluses that follow pressure blisters are the skin's way of adapting to new activities and preventing further injury.

• Guarding itself from drying out and cracking by producing an oily or waxy substance, called sebum, from many thousands of oil glands

Sebum is the skin's own natural moisturizer and softener. It prevents skin from drying out and losing its resiliency. Sebum also fights harmful bacteria that could cause infection. The glands that produce sebum are deep in the skin's inner layers. Many of them are attached to hair follicles. Blood provides the sebaceous glands with the acids, salts, fat, and water they need to manufacture sebum. A tiny amount of sebum is secreted at a steady rate. However, the amount varies in different parts of the body. The greatest supply is in the hairy areas. Too much or too little sebum makes the skin too dry or too oily, creating problems such as dandruff or acne.

• Taking in oxygen and giving off carbon dioxide

On a small scale but one that's essential to life, your skin performs the same function as your lungs by taking in oxygen and giving off carbon dioxide. In some cases, such as lung damage, the skin is capable of pitching in to aid in the work.

Scars, stretch marks, and keloids

Certain skin conditions are not disorders or diseases but natural, normal, and inevitable. These include scars, stretch marks, and keloids.

Scars

No one can avoid having one or more scars. Whether from cuts, burns, surgery, vaccinations, acne, or illnesses such as chicken pox, we all acquire them.

Scars have one thing in common: they're permanent. Time will cause them to lighten, thin out, or flatten but not to disappear entirely. A scar results from tissue repair. When this process occurs, the scar doesn't have the same makeup as the original, undamaged skin. Rubbing in any or all of a vast variety of ointments, creams, or oils is a waste of time, energy, and money. However, if a scar is very disfiguring or prominent, or if, for example, you're a movie star whose face must be seen on a giant screen, you may want to know about procedures that can be performed by a plastic surgeon or dermatologist to make a scar less conspic-

Scar

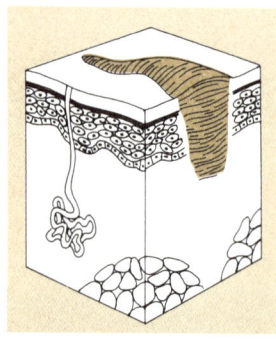

A scar is a mark on the skin that is left by the healing of injured tissue.

A newer implant

A newer "filler" called fibrel is currently being tested by the Food and Drug Administration (FDA). Fibrel, which is injected into the skin, combines gelatin, fibrin, other substances, and blood protein, Since the blood used is the patient's own, allergic reaction is unlikely. In addition, the benefits appear to be long-lasting.

uous. These include dermabrasion (planing down some layers of outer skin), chemosurgery, including acid treatments, and collagen implants.

• Dermabrasion

In dermabrasion, the skin is first "frozen" with a local anesthetic and then scraped with a rapidly rotating steel brush that has the effect of "leveling off" the surface. A treatment that takes about 20 minutes can produce a great improvement after the skin heals in a few weeks.

• Chemosurgery

With chemosurgery, a much more complicated procedure, various chemicals and acids create a more uniform appearance of the scarred or pitted area. A doctor must monitor any chemicals applied to the skin so that they don't work too quickly or penetrate too deeply and create damage at lower skin levels. (The goal is to remove outer layers of skin containing scars, wrinkles, or growths.) Usually, several sessions, scheduled over a period of weeks, are required. Chemosurgery is painful but the end result can give you smooth, firm skin in the formerly marred area.

• Collagen implants

In this treatment, collagen, a protein purified from cowhide, is injected under the skin to fill in and smooth out wrinkles, pock marks, acne scars, and other scars. There are two drawbacks to this treatment: some people are allergic to collagen, and the injections must be repeated regularly.

Stretch marks

This condition results from stretching of the skin over a period of months or years. Skin elasticity is destroyed.

Stretch marks are usually associated with pregnancy and obesity. However, weight lifters are also prone to them. Certain glandular disturbances and medicated ointments containing cortisone can also contribute to their formation. They occur most frequently on the abdomen, thighs, breasts, and hips. At first, due to inflammation, they appear as reddish or purplish lines, but they gradually turn white. As with any scars, stretch marks don't have the same tissue consistency as the rest of the skin.

Again, nothing applied to the skin (topically) will

Stretch mark

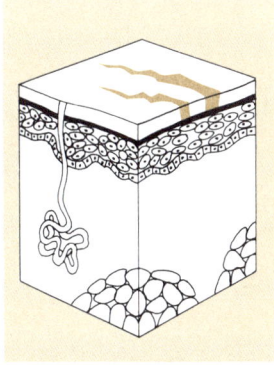

Stretch marks are reddish or purplish lines on the skin caused by loss of elasticity in the skin.

Keloid

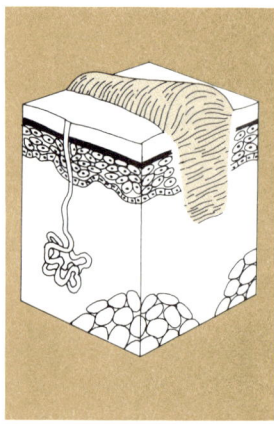

A keloid is an overgrowth of the healing fibrous tissue of the scar that causes a hard, slightly raised, reddened surface.

erase stretch marks. Only quite drastic surgery can be of any help.

To prevent stretch marks, avoid excessive weight gain during pregnancy and obesity at any time.

Keloids

Keloids are caused by injuries that, instead of healing, thicken and continue to thicken until they form a harmless growth. They appear as hard, smooth lumps. Keloids are more common in blacks and Orientals than in Caucasians, but the reason isn't understood.

It isn't a good idea to treat keloids unless they cause discomfort or are very large and unsightly because the treatment, whether by surgery, freezing, or X ray, isn't usually successful. Simple surgical removal of the keloid may lead to a new scar that thickens like the original keloid. Cortisone injections are sometimes used. Another treatment involves the injection of a cortisone-type suspension into the keloid. Freezing the keloid with dry ice or liquid nitrogen or using X ray therapy are other procedures. However, the older or larger the keloid, the less it responds to treatment.

2 Caring for your skin

Washing: good or bad?

Good as bathing and washing are, however, you can do too much of a good thing. Too much washing, particularly of aging skin that already has lost much of its natural lubrication, will deprive skin of sebum and oil and make it dry and flaky.

What's an acid mantle?

Our bodies have a natural covering called the acid mantle. It's composed of fatty acids from our perspiration and amino acids from our skin tissue. This acid mantle fights infection from bacteria that gather on the skin. The pH factor is a measurement of the percentage of hydrogen ions in the acid. The pH scale runs from 0 to 14, with 7 the neutral and ideal point.

Two basic actions can give you beautiful skin and prevent skin problems. First, practice proper hygiene, which simply means skin cleanliness; second, maintain good health with the help of proper nutrition and adequate exercise.

Proper skin hygiene

No fancy way of cleaning can do any more for your skin than what soap and water can. Your hard-working skin can't do its job if grime and grease clog its pores, its tiny surface openings.

Soap and water don't destroy the bacteria and viruses that become imbedded in and on your skin, but they do rinse these enemies off your skin and out of your pores. With the grease and dirt gone, you've taken step number one to protect your skin (and also to look more attractive).

Soap and water cleansing does more than make you look clean. When you take a bath or shower or wash your face and hands, flat, dry, dead skin cells, constantly sloughed off by the outer layer of the skin, are rinsed away. So is the outer layer of skin oil containing such debris as grime, soot, dust, toxic substances, and germs.

More sebum and perspiration will replace the washed off oil. If you make the water cooler at the end of the rinsing process, the skin may have a temporary tingly, revitalized feeling.

Older people, or people of any age with dry skin that doesn't produce adequate natural oil, will do better to wash with soaps, cleansing creams, or oils that preserve the skin's normal balance of acid and alkali, often called a neutral pH factor. These people may use soap only for dirtier areas.

The warmth of summer or exercise activates the sweat and sebaceous glands, covering the skin with natural oil. The situation is different in winter or cold climates. Cold air and heated indoor air dry skin. The skin's perspiration is reduced. The result is that too-frequent bathing, especially with soap, can produce dry, flaking, itching skin. How often is too often in the matter of bathing and soap usage is something that each individual will have to discover.

Soaps

What kind of soap should you select for your bath or shower? Today, we have a choice of hundreds of soaps, including superfatted (containing extra emollients), perfumed, hypoallergenic (containing no, or reduced, irritants, such as perfume), detergent. We have soaps for every purpose and every type of skin—oily, dry, allergic, alkaline, those with acne and other skin disorders. From over 100 available varieties of soap, we can buy a cake for 50 cents, $8.50, or much more.

You may opt for a plain soap or a fancy soap, but you want a personal soap that contains a minimum of alkali. This chemical substance neutralizes the acid on your skin and removes skin oil. Too much alkali can redden and irritate your skin. Also, modern soaps may have one or more chemical additives to disinfect your skin or to soften hard water; fats to create lavish suds; perfumes; colorings. Sensitive skin can suffer from almost any additive.

Guidelines for washing your face

1. Wet your face with warm water.

2. Use a soap or cleanser appropriate for your skin type.

3. Using your middle fingers, wash with upward and outward motions, except under your eyes.

4. Under your eyes, use light patting and gentle strokes from the outer corners toward your nose.

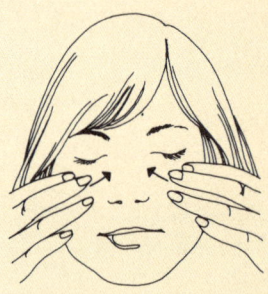

5. Rinse thoroughly with warm or cool water.

6. Pat dry.

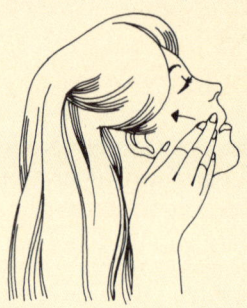

Some people require special soaps, such as acne soaps. Other people do well with soaps to which mild acids have been added. These acids counteract the alkaline quality of soap, making it match the normal skin mantle, pH7.

Some people have such extremely dry skin that they must avoid all soap or suffer chapping, itching, or flaking. Instead, they may prefer specially formulated "soapless" cleansers, cleansing creams, or oils.

Bath versus shower

Taking a shower may be preferable to taking a bath for the simple reason that dirt and soap are continuously and thoroughly rinsed away in the shower. However, many people prefer baths because they find them relaxing and soothing. In fact, one may, with the addition of fragrant oils, bubble bath, bath salts, and other sensory embellishments, transform a bath into a luxurious indulgence. In other cases, a physical problem, such as difficulty in standing or a condition like arthritis that requires a warm soak, may make a bath rather than a shower the appropriate or necessary choice.

Bath oils

Should you add bath oils to your bath water to counteract the drying tendency of soap? The chief advantage, aside from the pleasant psychological effect, is that the skin will feel smooth and silky. Also, bath oils provide brief relief for some skin conditions, such as contact dermatitis. (The oil forms a remoisturizing coating on the dry skin.)

These beneficial effects are only temporary. Why? Oils and creams applied on the skin's surface can't stimulate secretion of sebum, which is the true moisturizer and comes from within the skin. The moisturizer that we dunk ourselves in or cream on wears off or is sweated off, and our skin dries out again in a few hours.

Bath-oil risks

Another drawback to bath oils is that they're slippery: many people have suffered bad falls as a result of slipping on oily surfaces. What's more, bath oils make tubs harder to clean.

Facial care for healthy skin

The cosmetics industry is large, prosperous, and growing. Thousands of beauty preparations and cosmetics are offered and advertised in the most lavish, enticing, and expensive sales promotions. Their manufacturers are selling more than products. They're selling dreams—of beauty, youth, sexiness, and, of course, love.

An unpleasant surprise

Allergic reactions often take years to build up. Then, too, a manufacturer may change the ingredients in a product's formula, and you'd be unaware of it until too late.

Allergic reactions

Unfortunately, for many people, products meant to enhance attractiveness and a feeling of well-being may produce the opposite effect by causing very unattractive redness, swelling, pain, rashes, asthma, or eye irritations.

A vast array of chemicals goes into cosmetics, and you may be allergic to one. Determining the culprit can be a long and exasperating test of how good a detective you (and your doctor) are.

It's best, therefore, to stick with a product that has proven compatibility with your skin and chemistry. Sometimes, though, after many years of use, your tried-and-true product will turn on you, becoming an irritant and source of allergic reaction. If this occurs, seek medical treatment. On your own, you can try switching products, preferably to a hypoallergenic brand. These have the least amount of recognized allergens.

What's your skin type?

You can find selected cosmetics that will be beneficial to how you look and feel. Follow these procedures:

Determine your present skin type. Is it dry and sensitive, oily, or a combination of both? Your skin's characteristics may vary as you age or with a change in the seasons.

Test your skin type by washing your face with soap and water at bedtime and leaving off moisturizer. In the morning, normal skin should be smooth and have a light film of natural oil. Dry skin will feel tight; oily skin will be greasy; combination skin will have dry characteristics in one or more areas, such as the cheeks, and oily characteristics in others, usually the nose and forehead.

Clean skin is the starting point for healthy skin and also for beautiful skin. Depending on your skin type, cleanse your face with soap, cream, oil, or lotion.

Warning to sun worshippers

A sunburn damages the skin and may even cause a second-degree burn. Constant tanning will wrinkle and dry the skin and may result in skin cancers—it definitely leads to premature aging of exposed skin.

Face care guidelines

1. Soap is good for young or oily skin.

2. Cleansing cream can be used on any type of skin. Because it contains a good deal of oil, it's especially good to use a cleansing cream on dry skin. Remove the cream with tissues.

3. Cleansing oil is similar to but lighter than cleansing cream. It can also be used on all types of skin but is

A rule to remember
Whether cleansing, moisturizing, or applying makeup: always use upward and outward motions. The only exception is in the very delicate area under your eyes. Here, use light patting and very gentle strokes from the outer corner of your eye to the inner. This avoids unwanted stretching of the skin and muscles with resulting sagging and wrinkles.

Facial scrubs

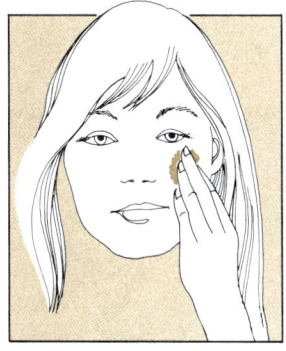

Some skin specialists say that washing with your usual soap or cleanser but using a washcloth each time produces the same results as occasional use of facial scrubs.

particularly suited for normal and oily skin. Some brands are less oily than others and can be rinsed off with water rather than tissued off. For many people, this gives cleansing oil a psychological advantage over cream.

4. Astringents and toners, with or without alcohol, should be used after the other cleansing methods. They remove any leftover cleanser from the skin.

Moisturizers
Moisturizing is a must. Air pollution, sun, wind, and cold all damage skin, even young people's skin. Therefore, all skin types, from childhood on, need moisturizing protection.

- The skin of very young people needs only a light moisturizer.

- Oily skins need a cream or lotion that is oil-free and can actually blot up excess oil.

- If you have acne or skin that is "broken out," use a medicated type of cream for the blemished areas and a different moisturizer for the others.

- In the large variety of available products, you'll find day creams, or moisturizers, and night creams. Day creams act to retain the skin's natural moisture and add additional moisture. They also serve as a silky base for makeup. If your skin is very dry, you'll need a heavier night cream for both day and night use.

- The dangers of exposing skin to the sun's rays are well recognized. Use a day cream that includes a sunscreen.

Facial scrubs
Facial scrubs (or exfoliators) are cream products containing an abrasive, or rough, substance. When massaged on freshly cleansed skin, they remove dead skin layers, stimulate circulation, help the skin absorb moisture from external sources, and leave it smoother and rosier. Depending on your skin type, use a scrub twice each week (oily skin) or every two weeks (dry skin). Always rinse the scrub off thoroughly and use a moisturizer afterward.

Facial masks
Facial masks come in two types: cleansing and peel-off. Both help to clean, tone, tighten, and **refresh** your skin by removing dead cells and stimulating circulation.

Facial masks

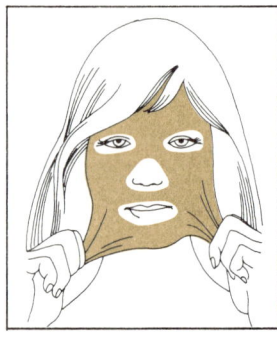

To get the most benefit from a facial mask, lie down (with your legs slightly elevated) and luxuriate. Afterward, your skin will look rosier, and you'll feel relaxed.

In addition to the steam
The herbal compound or oil will help open nasal passages.

Cleansing masks are thick creams that you smooth on. When they dry and harden, they must be softened with a warm, wet washcloth and then thoroughly rinsed off.

Peel-off masks are spread on, left to dry into a sort of "plastic skin," and then peeled (or washed) off.

Special masks are made for blemished skin and help to eliminate pimples and blackheads.

Steam
Steaming your face (every week or every other week for oily skin and once in 6 weeks for dry skin) can improve pore cleansing and, in the case of oily skin, help to get rid of pimples and blackheads.

1. Cleanse your face thoroughly and moisturize it well.
2. Pour an herbal compound or herbal oils in boiling water.
3. Lean over the steaming bowl or basin, and drape a towel over your head.

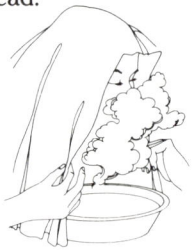

- If you prefer, allow the boiling water to cool sufficiently so that you can soak a towel in it, and then cover your face with the wrung-out towel as a hot compress.

- Steaming your face over boiling water should be done for no more than 10 minutes; the hot-compress method should be done for 2 or 3 minutes.

4. Afterward, rinse with cool water and blot your face dry.

Skin care for men
Basic masculine skin care has traditionally involved no more than washing and shaving. However, many men find aftershave lotion soothing to newly shaved skin, and some men enjoy wearing a pleasant fragrance.

Pharmaceutical companies have long competed with one another, offering shaving creams that are

Only one difference
Men's skin is no different from women's except for the portion under the eyes, which is less dry and sensitive in men than in women.

claimed to be "kinder" to a man's face. These products come in various consistencies and scents. Mentholated types are preferred by some men because they impart a soothing "coolness."

Cosmetics manufacturers recently have expanded their product lines to include a variety of skin care products for men. Among these are facial scrubs (exfoliators), moisturizers, and bronzers. Bronzers are actually a form of makeup intended to provide a robust, healthy-looking color.

Hair removal for women

The growth of unwanted hair causes much unhappiness. Fortunately, getting rid of unwanted hair is no problem at all compared to trying to grow hair, replace it, or transplant it.

Although excessive hairiness may be the result of a glandular dysfunction, requiring medical treatment or surgery, superfluous hair usually results from our internal makeup. And the latter may, at some point, undergo a change, such as during a stressful period or menopause (which produces hormonal imbalances).

There are six ways to remove hair:

Abrasion

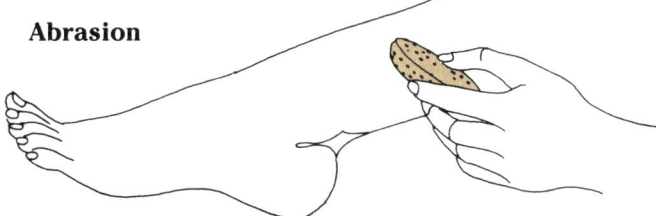

Abrasion uses specially constructed flat round discs and pumice stones to rub hair away. As with shaving, only surface hair is removed. Abrasion is slower and more irritating than shaving and is more apt to lead to infection.

Plucking

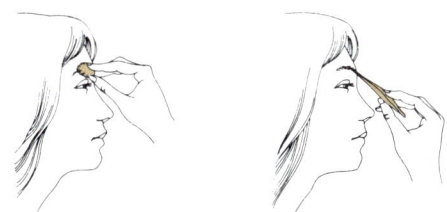

Plucking with tweezers is the most common method of hair removal. Many people pluck hair from eyebrows

More hair

When we grow superfluous hair, we aren't growing additional hairs. The number of hairs we were born with remains the same. However, we have two types of hair: the long and thick, and the short, almost invisible type. When we become overly hairy, the short, "peach fuzz" variety increases in length and thickness.

and other facial areas. Plucking won't make hairs grow in thicker and coarser. First, swab the area to be plucked with alcohol to prevent infection in the openings left by the pulled-out hairs. Sterilize the tweezers, too. Work in a good light with a magnifying mirror.

Shaving

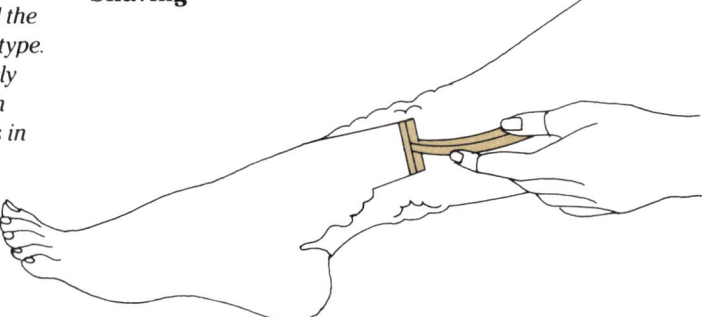

Shaving is a popular method for removing hair from larger areas such as legs. Unlike plucking, shaving does not remove hairs from beneath the surface but only cuts them off. Therefore, the procedure must be repeated frequently, approximately every second or third day. Using warm water and a shaving cream will reduce irritation and help avoid nicks and cuts. If these do occur, use an antiseptic to prevent infection in the opened skin area. (Shaving doesn't increase hair growth, but it does produce stubble, and new hair may appear darker.)

Chemical depilatories

Chemical depilatories are quite popular. Various preparations, in cream or lotion form, are applied to the skin. These are later washed or scraped off, removing hair with greater or lesser efficiency. Relatively painless, a depilatory delays re-growth for about 10 days because it penetrates into the hair follicle. Depilatories contain chemicals, so you should test a small skin area for allergic reaction. If there isn't any, the hairy area should be washed and dried and the chemical applied according to directions. Afterward, cleanse the treated area thoroughly and apply a soothing cream. Never use a chemical depilatory on a skin area that is cut or scraped.

A few drawbacks

Using a wax depilatory is somewhat painful and irritating to the skin. Also, the follicles may be damaged, which may cause thicker regrowth.

Wax depilatories

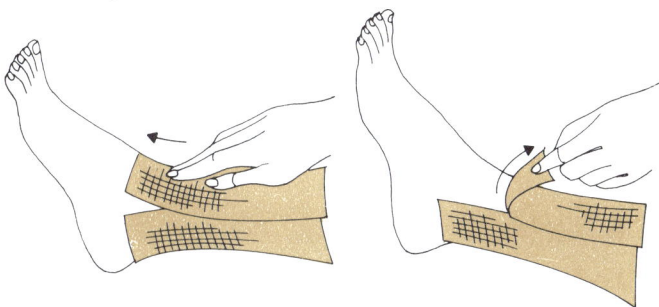

Wax depilatories are of two types. One is used at room temperature (as it comes from the jar or tube) and is rather hard to spread. The other variety must be heated into a warm, sticky paste. With either type, the skin should be washed and dried first. Then the wax is applied and strips of cloth are pressed over it. When the recommended time has elapsed, you yank off the strips—the wax and hair are thus yanked off the skin. (Yank in the opposite direction of hair growth.) This method tears the hairs away from their follicles, leaving the skin free of hair for approximately 4 weeks.

The skin should be thoroughly washed afterward and a soothing cream applied.

Permanent hair removal

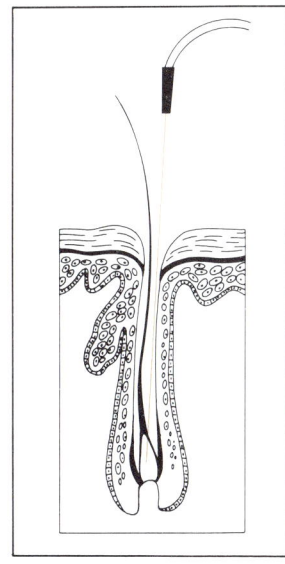

Performed properly by a skilled technician, electrolysis removes hair permanently. However, electrolysis involves time. Clearing large areas on arms and legs can take a few years of weekly or twice-weekly sessions. It's also expensive and uncomfortable.

Electrolysis

Electrolysis, the most effective method of hair removal, can be painful, expensive, and time-consuming. If done properly by a licensed electrologist or dermatologist, electrolysis removes hair permanently, without scars, and the skin may be smoother than before.

In electrolysis, a thin platinum or stainless steel needle is inserted into one hair follicle at a time. The operator traces each hair shaft until the tip of the needle reaches the papilla, also called the hair bulb, around the hair root. (Care is taken not to puncture the hair shaft itself as this could result in scarring.) Next, the operator uses electric current to destroy the hair root. Another hair can't grow from a dead root. Each treated hair is pulled from its follicle with tweezers. An electrolysis session usually lasts for a half-hour, during which time about 50 hairs are removed. The amount of hair to be removed and the efficiency of the treatment will determine the number of sessions required.

Scalp care

We've all seen TV commercials promoting shiny, lustrous hair with "bounce" and "body." And we've all heard about hair being a person's "crowning glory." Having hair become dry, brittle, or thin can be a distressing experience.

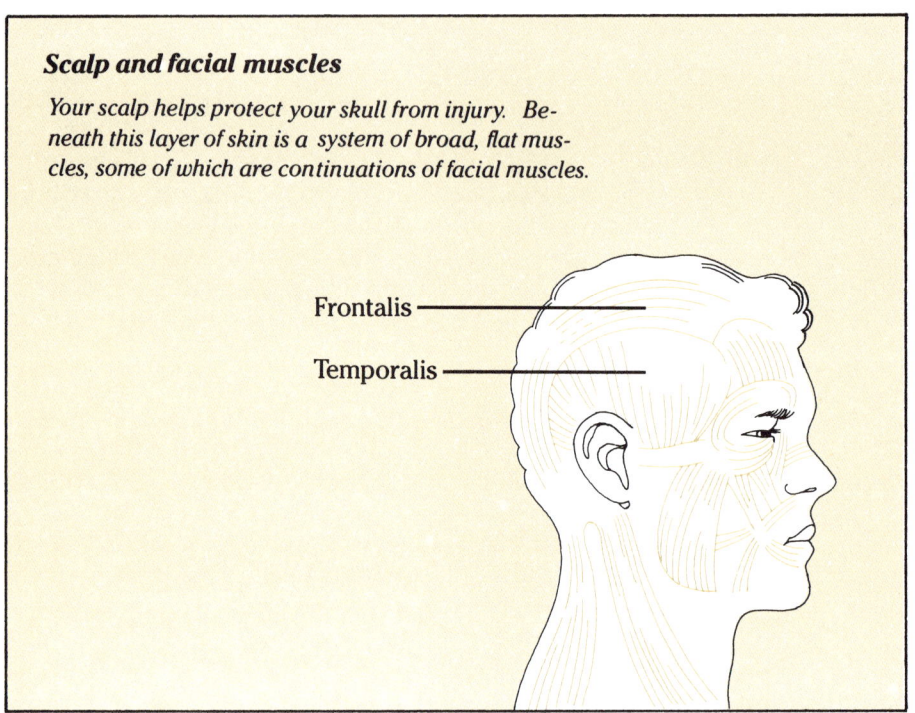

Scalp and facial muscles

Your scalp helps protect your skull from injury. Beneath this layer of skin is a system of broad, flat muscles, some of which are continuations of facial muscles.

Frontalis

Temporalis

What can you do to protect or promote a head full of healthy hair? Proper scalp care is a vital course of action. Just as you wouldn't (or shouldn't) allow grime, dust, grease, toxic substances, or germs to accumulate on your face or other areas of your skin, neither should you let your scalp, a part of your skin, be dirty and neglected. Follow these suggestions:

• Shampoo regularly

Contrary to a common and false belief, frequent shampooing will not wash away the essential oils necessary for healthy hair and scalp. What will be washed away is dirt. Young people's hair or oily hair at any age should be shampooed daily or at least 3 times a week. Dry hair should be shampooed at least once a week. Use a shampoo and comfortably warm water to help loosen whatever dirt or grease is on your scalp or in your hair. Rinse the shampoo off thoroughly.

- Brush

Brushing your hair can help keep it clean and can stimulate your scalp. But the old rule of "100 strokes a day" has been repealed. We now recognize that brushing an oily scalp spreads grease throughout the hair. Also, too frequent or too vigorous brushing can cause the opposite effects: dryness of the scalp caused by removing needed sebum, and broken hair caused by too much pulling and stroking. When you comb and brush your hair, use a natural bristle brush and hard rubber comb. Wash your brush and comb after each use.

- Massage your scalp

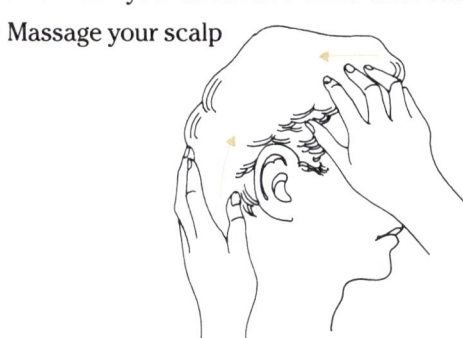

Massage your scalp frequently to stimulate circulation and oil production. Use your fingertips in stroking motions backward from your forehead and upward from the base of your neck.

- Don't pull your hair

Avoid pulling on your hair when it's wet or dry, whether during massaging or by wearing "stretching" hairstyles. Slow but steady hair loss and an increasingly "high forehead" will result from the strain on the hair.

- Don't interfere with circulation

Don't interfere with good circulation in your scalp by wearing anything tight—hats, headbands, or wigs.

- Don't let your scalp become too dry

If your scalp is dry, apply a vegetable oil (such as olive, castor, or peanut) as often as necessary to keep it soft and pliable. Some people find that warming the oil first and leaving it on for an hour under a plastic cap produces excellent results. Be sure to shampoo thoroughly after the oil treatment.

- Eat a healthful diet

A healthful diet is as essential for the health of your scalp as it is for the health of the rest of your body.

Do dandruff shampoos work?
Commercially available dandruff shampoos don't make distinctions among the scalp conditions that can cause dandruff. What's worse, if overused by a dandruff victim, many of these shampoos can cause flaking of their own. If you have a mild case of dandruff, the best shampoo to use is a simple soap shampoo without harsh antidandruff detergents. If your dandruff is persistent and bothersome, see a dermatologist.

Dandruff

Dandruff is both the most obvious and the most common scalp problem. In fact, in some degree, it's a universal condition.

All over the skin's surface, new cells are constantly replacing dead ones. The used-up cells move to the skin's surface and flake off.

If excessive, this process can create a scalp condition requiring attention or medical treatment. Dandruff is a disorder of the sebaceous glands and can occur if the scalp is either too oily or too dry. Excessive sebum production causes the scalp to scale into flakes of dead skin. Underproduction of sebum causes the scalp to become so dry that the growth of its top layer is accelerated and breaks off into flakes.

Other factors can promote dandruff: bacteria or fungi on your scalp, incomplete rinsing off of shampoo, improper diet, emotional stress, infection, or hormonal imbalances.

While it isn't life-threatening, dandruff is unattractive and extremely unpopular.

Take these actions:

1. Keep your scalp clean.
2. Brush your hair and scalp with a natural bristle brush before shampooing to loosen skin flakes.
3. Shampoo frequently, thoroughly, and correctly. Be sure to remove every trace of shampoo with thorough rinsing.
4. Even if your scalp is itchy, don't scratch it with your fingernails. The result can be an infection that will compound the problem.
5. If your dandruff persists, consult a dermatologist, who will probably prescribe special scalp medication, shampoo, dietary changes, or other procedures.

An FDA warning
A Food and Drug Administration (FDA) panel studied dandruff shampoos. The panel warned that such products should be kept out of the eyes or rinsed out quickly if they get in; should not be used on children under 2 except as directed by a doctor; and should be kept out of the reach of all children, since some of the ingredients in these products are poisonous if ingested.

Diet for beautiful skin

Like any of your other organs, your skin requires adequate and appropriate nourishment. Skin cells need the same nutrients other body cells need to manufacture new cells, metabolize energy, and fight disease. A healthy skin is the result of what goes from your mouth to your digestive tract to your bloodstream.

The food you eat puts the required nutrients into your bloodstream through your body's digestive and metabolic processes. Passing through your arteries and tiny capillaries, blood delivers nutrients to your skin. The blood then returns through your capillaries and veins, removing waste material.

Diet and acne

The connection between diet and acne has become a controversial issue. Dermatologists aren't as strict about diet as they were in former years, but many still recommend cutting down, as far as possible, on fatty foods such as milk, butter, ice cream, French-fried potatoes, salad dressing, mayonnaise, potato chips, peanut butter, pizza, and chocolate. Diet has become less stressed in acne treatment because now we know that the disorder results from a variety of factors.

In general, fresh foods, properly prepared—raw, if appropriate—moderate in amount, low in fat and sugar content, high in vitamin and mineral content, promote healthy skin and a healthy body.

Although certain substances applied to the skin (such as Vitamin A ointment for acne) may be beneficial, the skin's ability to function depends primarily upon what you put inside your body, rather than what you put on the exterior.

Recommended Dietary Allowances (RDA)

Beautiful skin is only one of the many benefits of a balanced diet. The easiest way to make certain your meals are filling your vitamin and mineral needs is to follow the established RDAs.

Protein, quality equal to or greater than casein, a high-quality milk protein .... 45 grams (g.)
quality less than casein .... 65 g.

Vitamin A ...... 5,000 International Units (I.U.)
Vitamin C .... 60 milligrams (mg.)
Thiamine (Vitamin B_1) .... 1.5 mg.
Riboflavin (Vitamin B_2) .... 1.7 mg.
Niacin (Vitamin B_3) .... 20 mg.
Calcium .... 1.0 g.
Iron .... 18 mg.
Vitamin D .... 400 I.U.
Vitamin E .... 30 I.U.
Vitamin B_6 .... 2.0 mg.
Folic acid (Folate, folacin) .... 0.4 mg.
Vitamin B_{12} .... 6 micrograms (mcg.)
Phosphorous .... 1.0 g.
Iodine .... 150 mcg.
Magnesium .... 400 mg.
Zinc .... 15 mg.
Copper .... 2 mg.
Biotin .... 0.3 mg.
Pantothenate (Pantothenic acid) .... 10 mg.

Skin disorders and vitamin deficiencies

Certain skin disorders are directly related to vitamin deficiencies. For example:

- Vitamin A

Insufficiency of Vitamin A can produce dryness, roughness, or splotchy marks on the skin. Vitamin A is supplied in yellow fruits, vegetables such as spinach and broccoli, liver, butter, and fish-liver oil such as cod liver oil.

- Vitamin B complex

A Vitamin B-complex deficiency can result in cracked lips, scaling of the skin, and dermatitis. One component of the Vitamin B complex—niacin—is linked to pellagra, a disorder characterized by skin rashes. Good sources of Vitamin B are liver, whole grain cereals, including wheat germ, dark green leafy vegetables, poultry, fish, and nutritional yeast.

- Vitamin C

A Vitamin C deficiency may be marked by bleeding gums or red spots around sweat pores and hair follicles. Vitamin C, found in citrus fruits, berries, peppers, leafy greens, and cabbage, can aid in wound healing because it's linked to the formation of collagen, the body's glue that fills in the tissues and literally holds us together.

- Vitamin D

A Vitamin D deficiency undermines bone health. This vitamin can be manufactured from sunlight on the skin. It's found in fish such as sardines, herring, salmon, cod and cod liver oil, as well as egg yolks and liver.

- Vitamin E

While Vitamin E deficiency is rare, this vitamin helps to heal skin ulcerations and other skin disorders. It also protects the skin's various functions. Combined with Vitamin A, Vitamin E is proving effective in combatting acne.

If you suspect that your meals are not supplying you with adequate nutrition, you may want to use over-the-counter one-a-day-type multivitamin and mineral supplements. For additional vitamin and mineral supplementation, consult your doctor.

Skin and weight problems

Staying within your normal weight is important to skin health. Being overweight can lead to skin problems in the form of chafing, irritation, and stretch marks. And crash dieting can be responsible for wrinkling, sagging, and loss of skin tone.

3

Skin emergencies

Sites unseen
Burns resulting from explosions can cause unseen damage to lungs (the result of breathing excessively hot air), and electric burns (including being struck by lightning) can have injurious effects on the heart and respiration. Internal burns can result from several causes, such as accidentally swallowing an acid—lye, for example—that burns the esophagus.

Accidents can occur any time, anywhere. While we can't predict them and often can't prevent them, we can be prepared to deal with them. Any trauma (damage) to the skin, whether major or minor, requires immediate attention and care. The more severe cases require prompt professional treatment.

Burns

Each year in the United States, 2 million people suffer burns. When a large skin area is affected, it constitutes a life-threatening injury. Such cases require immediate medical treatment at specialized burn centers or hospitals with trauma units.

The most immediate dangers of burns are shock and infection. The shock that results from injury results in circulatory disturbance and is marked by lowered blood pressure, rapid pulse, clammy and pale skin, anxiety, or unconsciousness.

Because a burn destroys the body's protective covering, the function of the skin to act as our body's thermostat is lost.

In addition, the destroyed skin can no longer prevent the loss of vital body fluids; nor can it act as a barrier against harmful bacteria. Because nerve endings have been destroyed, the skin can't relay information to the brain. In this condition, it's also unable to protect our inner organs.

Although we tend to think that burns result only from contact with heat—fire, sun, boiling water, for example—they can also be caused by contact with certain chemicals or excessive cold that leads to frostbite.

Burns are painful, but deep burns can actually be less painful than superficial ones because of the destruction of nerve endings. It's a paradox that a person suffering very intense burn pain may be less seriously injured than one with less pain.

With a little first-aid treatment, minor burns will heal themselves. However, deeper burns can be life-threatening, even fatal. The degree of danger related to a burn depends upon its depth. For this reason, burns have been classified into degrees.

First-degree-burn depth

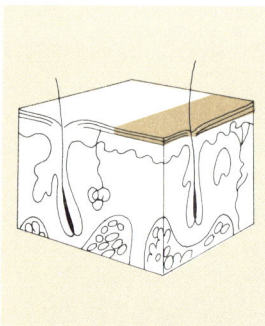

Sometimes too much sun can produce a first-degree burn, which includes reddening and swelling of the skin.

Second-degree-burn depth

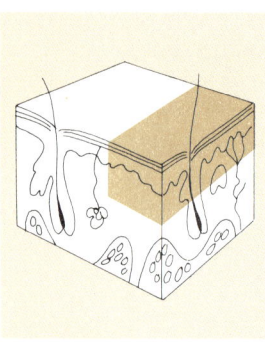

Second-degree burns are more serious, producing blisters that may be either superficial or deep. Such burns can usually heal themselves.

First-degree burns

First-degree burns are superficial. They may be very painful, and the skin becomes red, but they're self-healing and usually don't leave scars. A mild sunburn is an example of this type of burn.

First aid:

1. Apply cold water compresses to the affected area or submerge it in cold water. This should relieve some of the pain. If you apply the cold the moment you're burned, you'll actually stop tissue damage.

2. Apply a dry dressing. Never apply antiseptic ointments of any kind to a burn—they will only make the condition worse.

The juice of the aloe vera plant or ointments made from this substance as well as the form of Vitamin B known as pantothenic acid have proved not only to relieve the pain of burns but to assist healing.

Second-degree burns

Second-degree burns are not only extremely reddened and blistered but are severe enough to extend into deeper skin layers, damaging capillaries, sweat glands, and hair follicles. This results in the leakage of fluid from the blood (plasma) into surrounding tissue. Although painful, these burns, too, are usually capable of healing themselves. The deeper cells are not too damaged to regenerate new skin, and, depending on the type of skin affected, there is little or no scarring.

However, if a very large area is involved, the person may suffer greatly. A very severe sunburn, contact with a hot stove burner, or having a hot liquid spilled on you are examples of this type of burn.

First aid:

Second-degree burns usually require medical care. However, you can treat some, such as severe sunburns, yourself. Follow these guidelines:

1. Immerse the burned area in cold water.
2. Apply a dry dressing.
3. Blisters should not be broken; tissue should not be removed.
4. If possible, keep the affected area higher than the heart.
5. Drink as much fluid as possible.
6. Use aspirin or an aspirin substitute to relieve pain.

Third-degree-burn depth

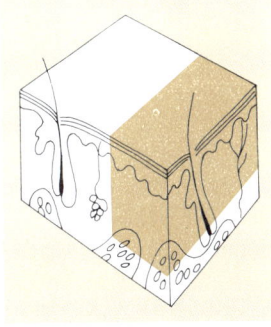

Third-degree burns are potentially life-threatening. Besides destroying the entire skin, fat, muscle, even bone may be burned, and scarring is unavoidable.

Skin grafts
The very latest advance in grafting is the technique of growing sheets of a victim's skin from a very small piece of skin taken from the body. This near-miracle results from a tissue culture utilizing a small patch of undamaged skin.

Third-degree burns

Third-degree burns may involve destruction through all layers of the skin. They may even result in white or charred appearance of the skin. The cells that could regenerate new skin have been destroyed, and skin grafting is required. Very severe burns must be treated at a hospital or burn center that provides highly specialized intensive care. A third-degree burn might be produced if your clothing caught fire and the flames were not extinguished immediately.

First aid:
Third-degree burns require immediate medical attention.

1. As an emergency measure, shock should be combatted by giving the conscious patient fluids to drink and having the patient lie down (with feet raised).
2. Cover the burned area with clean wrappings.
3. Arrange transportation to a hospital immediately.

Burn treatment

A burn's severity may not be fully known for several days. The symptoms—redness, blistering, charring, pain—must be evaluated as they develop. However, with all burns, the dangers of shock and infection must be dealt with from the start.

In the past 25 years, medical science has made marvelous progress in saving burn victims from death and disfigurement. Previously, a nonlethal burn could become lethal because of infection. New creams, antibiotics, intravenous solutions to compensate for fluid loss or to replace it, and the use of radioactive gas to detect lung burns are some of the medical milestones that have cut the death rate from serious burns.

- Skin grafts

Skin grafting involves the replacement of damaged skin with healthy skin. Grafting preserves vital body functions, such as heat control, and prevents fluid loss. Skin for grafting is usually taken from the victim's thigh, back, or abdomen (new skin grows over the area from which the graft is taken). If a burn victim cannot provide skin for a graft, skin from family members, a volunteer donor, or a cadaver may be used. In some cases, even pigskin has been used as a graft.

However, the body's immune system causes rejection of foreign invaders, including most grafts. The possibility of rejection is least when the victim's own skin is used. That of an identical twin is second best, followed by the skin of a family member. A cadaver's skin will be rejected in a few weeks and pigskin in one week. Yet the gained time may save the victim's life.

Chemical burns

Chemical burns are similar to fire burns in that not only your skin but your underlying tissues can be damaged. The chemicals most often involved are acids and alkalis, such as turpentine, lye, nitric acid, and paint remover. Many household cleaning agents contain chemicals that will burn skin. The severity of skin damage depends on several factors: how large an area of skin is involved; how long the chemical remains on the skin before being washed off; the strength and concentration of the chemical.

First aid:

Chemical burns require immediate medical care.

1. Flush the area with large amounts of water.

2. Remove or cut away contaminated clothing and remove jewelry.

3. Contact a doctor, emergency room, or poison control center immediately for specific instructions.

Frostbite

Frostbite is similar to a burn in the sense that skin damage and injury to underlying tissue can result. The difference is that frostbite is caused by the freezing of a body part, such as ears, nose, fingers, or toes.

When a body surface is exposed to extremely cold air or fluids, the blood vessels beneath constrict so drastically that blood supply is cut off from surface areas. These areas may then freeze. Deprived of blood circulation, heat, and moisture, the frozen tissue begins to die. In the most severe cases, infection, ulceration, and gangrene of the affected part can result. Amputation may be necessary.

Frostbite symptoms are tingling, burning, and pain. The skin may initially turn a bluish shade. When feeling has been totally lost, the skin becomes waxy white or grayish yellow. Blisters may appear.

First aid:

Remember that as the affected area thaws, intense pain will develop.

Frostbite first aid

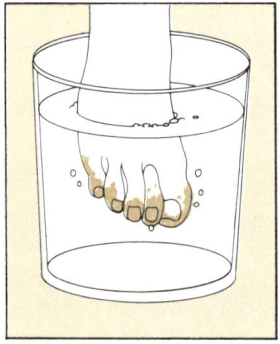

The first thing to do for frostbite is soak the frozen area in warm (102 to 105 degrees F.) — not hot — water.

Wash hands first
Remember to wash your hands before treating any injury.

1. The frozen area should be soaked in warm (102 to 105 degrees F.)—not hot—water. If this is not feasible, thaw the frozen part with the person's own body heat (such as placing a hand in an armpit) or with another person's body heat. Cover the victim with towels or blankets.

2. Don't rub or massage the frozen area and don't apply snow, ice, or ice water as these measures may increase the injury.

3. Give hot drinks (coffee, tea, soup)—as much as the victim can drink—to restore warmth and help dilate the blood vessels.

4. Aspirin or a substitute will relieve pain during the thawing process.

5. Do not break blisters.

6. Arrange transportation to a hospital immediately.

Abrasion

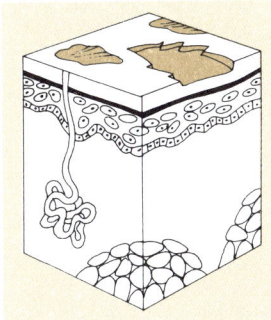

Abrasions

Abrasions are superficial injuries, such as a skinned knee, caused by rubbing away the top layer of the skin. Bleeding from an abrasion is slight, but a pinkish fluid may ooze from the injured area.

Because the protective skin covering has been removed, nerve endings are exposed, and pain results.

First aid:

1. As with a cut, gently clean the area with warm water and soap. Hydrogen peroxide is helpful, too. Pat the area dry.

2. Do not scrub an abrasion as this will do further damage and cause additional pain.

3. Coat the injured area with an antibacterial ointment.

4. If coarse bits of dirt don't wash off, remove them gently with tweezers.

5. If the damage is not too severe, leave the abrasion exposed to air. If it's too large an area or too irritated, cover it loosely (allowing air to circulate) with clean (preferably sterile) gauze or cloth and fasten with adhesive tape.

Cleaning an abrasion
If you must use tweezers to remove particles from an abrasion, boil the tweezers for 10 minutes, or sterilize them in the flame of several matches and wipe the carbon away with sterile gauze.

6. If the injury can't be properly cleaned with this basic care, medical attention is required and perhaps a tetanus immunization.

Cuts

Cuts (or lacerations) are open wounds. The skin is "sliced" or torn, and the injury may extend into the underlying skin tissue. Pain and often profuse bleeding can result.

First aid:

1. Clean the cut or laceration thoroughly with warm running water and soap. In addition to reducing bacteria that could cause infection, this procedure should help to remove any bits of glass, gravel, or grease that have become imbedded in the skin. An antiseptic solution such as hydrogen peroxide will aid in this cleansing process.

2. Control bleeding by covering the wound with

How the skin heals

The skin protects the body from infection, and any injury to the skin is healed rapidly to restore this protective barrier.

The moment the skin is cut, the broken capillary blood vessels constrict to stop the flow of blood out of the body and to prevent germs from entering the body. The capillary blood vessels open again to release substances that cause clotting. One clotting substance is the blood protein fibrin. Fibrin makes up very fine threads of protein that bring the edges of the wound together. These threads eventually cover the entire

Unbroken skin

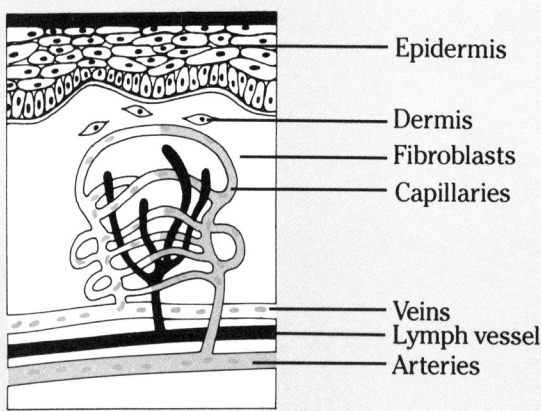

The internal parts of the body are protected by the skin.

Skin with a cut

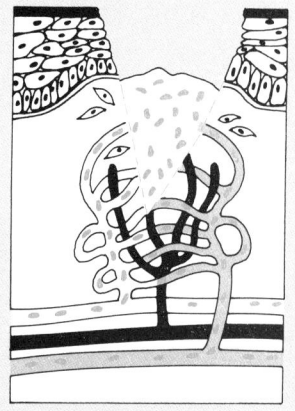

Any injury to the skin can expose the body to infection.

sterile gauze or the cleanest cloth available, held in place by a bandage or adhesive tape. Apply pressure to the bandage to slow bleeding and maintain the pressure until professional help is available.

Deep cuts or lacerations may require stitches (sutures) to complete the closing of the wound and reduce scarring. A professional examination is important to determine if damage has been done to nerves, tendons, or the large blood vessels located beneath the skin. The victim may also need a tetanus immunization.

wound and harden into a scab. Beneath the scab healing can take place.

Shortly after an injury to the skin, white blood cells begin to break down and remove bacteria, debris, and other foreign matter from the wound. In the inner layer of the skin, cells called fibroblasts move into the wound and form new tissue.

In the outer layer, the epidermal cells reproduce to form new skin. When this new layer of skin is completed, the scab falls off, leaving little sign of the injury.

One day later

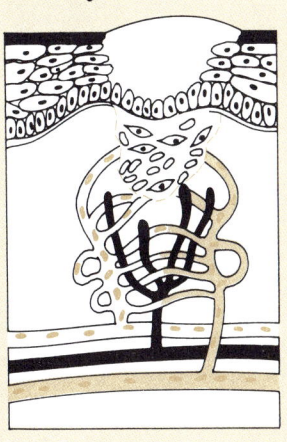

The cut is beginning to heal.

Two days later

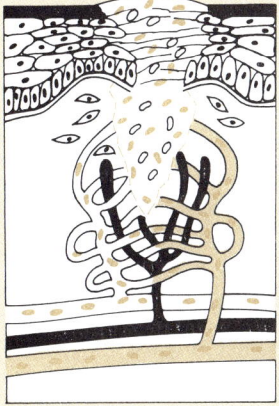

New tissue replaces the injured skin.

One week later

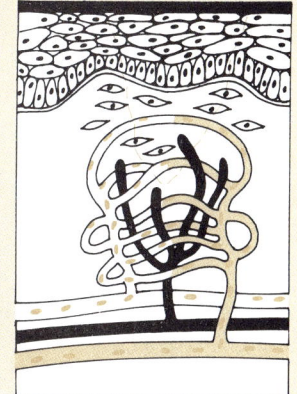

New tissue continues to grow under a protective scab.

4

Acne

Where acne appears

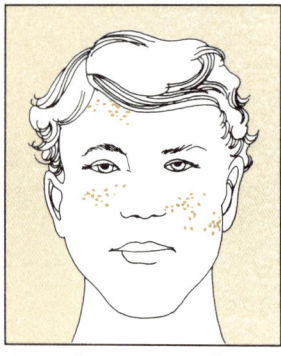

Acne often appears along the hairline, on the cheeks, and sometimes on the chin. Acne doesn't always confine itself to the face; it can appear on the upper back and shoulders, upper arms, and chest.

Acne has been called the plague of adolescence. The National Center for Health Statistics reports that only 27.7 percent of Americans between the ages of 12 and 17 escape having acne. That leaves nearly three-quarters of our nation's adolescents suffering acne.

Nor is acne limited to teenagers. Adults, too, can have this disfiguring and scarring disease. Sometimes people who've had beautiful skin for two or three decades suddenly begin to "break out" in their twenties or thirties.

Causes of acne

Hormonal production during adolescence is thought to be the primary contributing factor to acne. The amounts of hormones produced vary, and this imbalance sets the stage for overproduction of skin oils. The glands that produce skin oils become enlarged and clogged with excess oil, or sebum. Whiteheads and blackheads form.

As the oil builds up and is trapped, bacteria multiply. Acne thrives in the areas where there is the greatest number of oil glands—particularly on the face.

Several other factors can contribute to or cause acne:

- Oil and grease

Any oil or grease that comes in contact with the skin and further plugs the overloaded and overactive oil glands or causes excess sebum production will aggravate acne. Some sources of unwanted additional grease include improperly cleansed skin, long hair, "bangs" on the forehead, or oil and grease that get on the skin at work (in the garage, kitchen, workshop, factory).

- Medications

The use of certain drugs and medications, such as oral contraceptives, cortisones, iodides, bromides, and drugs used to control seizures, can cause or worsen acne.

A whitehead

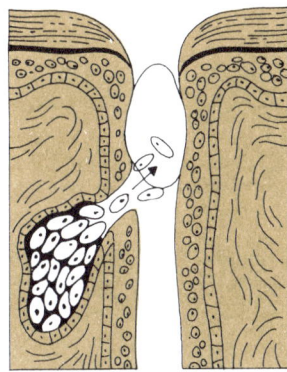

Sebum is produced by the sebaceous glands. Sometimes sebum plugs up a pore and becomes a whitehead pimple.

A blackhead

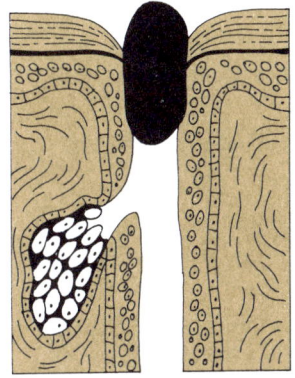

A blackhead forms after sebum has plugged up a pore and dead skin cells have accumulated.

- Fluoride

Fluoride-containing toothpastes have been observed to trigger acne around the mouth.

- Emotional stress

Emotional stress may aggravate the condition.

- Diet

The long-held belief that certain foods are a major cause of acne has been largely discredited by recent studies. However, many dermatologists still recommend avoidance of the traditional "no-nos"—chocolate, sugar, fried foods (especially French fries), oily foods (especially peanut butter), iodized salt, dairy products (such as milk and cheese), and shellfish. Sebaceous glands may become additionally overproductive when stimulated by these foods.

Symptoms of acne

Acne is an inflammation of the sebaceous (oil) glands located just beneath the skin's surface. This inflammation causes eruptions on the skin, usually on the face but in some cases on the neck, back, shoulders, chest, and arms. These eruptions—often called pimples, whiteheads, blackheads, or "zits"—appear as raised, red swellings. Many of these have little pockets of pus at their centers. Whiteheads and blackheads and, in severe cases, boils, cysts, and abscesses are present. Frequently, scarring of the skin (pits) remains long after the active symptoms have disappeared.

Most cases of acne disappear by the early twenties. However, the scars can be permanent. Those on the skin may be treated by surgery and other methods. Unfortunately, the emotional scars that remain are difficult to deal with.

Treatment for acne

Take the following actions to prevent or treat acne:

- Washing

Keeping the skin thoroughly clean is essential.

- Ointments

Applying antibacterial ointments to the affected skin areas controls the pus-forming germs that aggravate acne.

- Soaps and cleansers

Using specially medicated soaps, cleansers, astringents, and oil-free cosmetics can be helpful.

Tretinoin precaution
Using tretinoin requires special care. Follow your doctor's instructions and these precautions:

Never put tretinoin on wet skin—it'll penetrate much faster and cause problems.

Be careful about going out in the sun while using tretinoin—the chances of becoming severely burned are greatly increased by the medication's sensitizing action.

Don't use astringent cleansers—they can irritate the sensitive skin.

Accutane precaution
Women should take every precaution to avoid becoming pregnant while taking Accutane. Many doctors require female patients to take pregnancy tests before beginning Accutane treatment and urge them to use birth-control methods during treatment.

- Vitamins

The B-complex vitamins help to reduce oiliness and arrest blackhead formation; Vitamin C helps prevent infections and the spread of acne; Vitamin E aids in preventing scarring.

- Diet

Avoiding fatty foods is sometimes helpful in controlling acne.

If your acne is serious and resists your efforts, you'll want to see a doctor. Doctors use several methods of treating acne, among them:

- Antibiotics

The use of antibiotics such as tetracycline or erythromycin (given first by mouth and later applied to the skin) is an effective treatment.

- Tretinoin

Probably the best acne treatment involves tretinoin, a prescription medication available under the brand names Retin-A and Aberel. Tretinoin works by producing peeling and drying of the skin. Pimples are sloughed off, and any developing pimples are brought to the surface and dried up.

Tretinoin is available as both a cream and liquid; it's usual to begin treatment with the cream.

This medication requires patience—it may take two or three months before your skin begins to clear.

- Accutane

The drug Accutane, taken orally, has proven effective in the treatment of acne. Four to five months of treatment with the medication clears the complexion completely for more than 80 percent of patients, and this improvement is often permanent.

Accutane is expensive and can have bad side effects. Many users experience chapped lips, eye irritation, facial redness, muscular aches, and joint pain. These side effects end when treatment stops. The most serious problem with Accutane is birth defects in children of women who become pregnant while taking the drug.

- Natural Vitamin A

Natural Vitamin A (in water-soluble form), particularly when combined with zinc, has a beneficial effect on skin and may alleviate acne. Your doctor must advise you about the proper dosages.

Comedone extractor

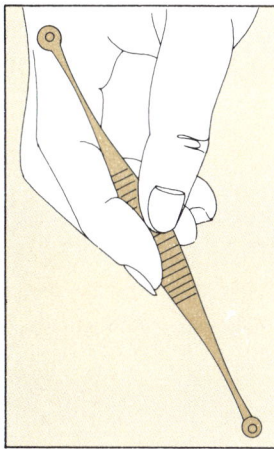

Squeezing pimples is never a good idea. Bacteria and infection may spread, causing new pimples to form and possibly causing scars. Never use a comedone extracor. If you have a pimple that is painful or that you think needs to be drained, see your dermatologist.

• Ultraviolet treatment
Ultraviolet treatment may be useful by producing a peeling of the outer skin layer, thereby allowing the plugged pores to empty.

• Injections
In the most severe cases, injections of cortisone or steroids, cryotherapy (temporary freezing of the skin), collagen injections, or surgery may be necessary.

Prevention of acne

Follow the general rules for proper skin care and follow these guidelines:

• Keep your skin very clean by gently washing it several times a day.

• Keep your hair and scalp clean by shampooing as often as advisable.

• Wear a hairstyle that keeps your hair off your face.

• Don't use oily cosmetics and moisturizers (unless you have very dry skin).

• Don't squeeze or pick pimples or blackheads. Doing so may spread bacteria and infection and scar your skin.

• Maintain good nutrition. Avoid greasy, oil-saturated foods; keep your vitamin and mineral intake at an adequate level.

• Avoid stress and emotional upset. Worry and irritation don't usually help a troubling situation, and they can make things worse by adding a skin problem to your other worries.

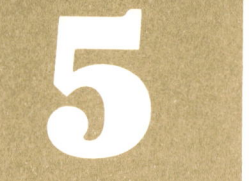

Sunburn and sun poisoning

Trying to acquire a suntan is the most common way of becoming sunburned. It's a dangerous process. We may want to look golden, tawny, bronzed, and healthy; instead, we may end up with burned, reddened, blistered skin that's painful and unattractive. The long-range effect is to make us look prematurely old—wrinkled, discolored, saggy, and leathery. All of these sun-caused problems are irreversible—no treatment can repair the damage once it's done. Worst of all, we're encouraging the development of skin cancer.

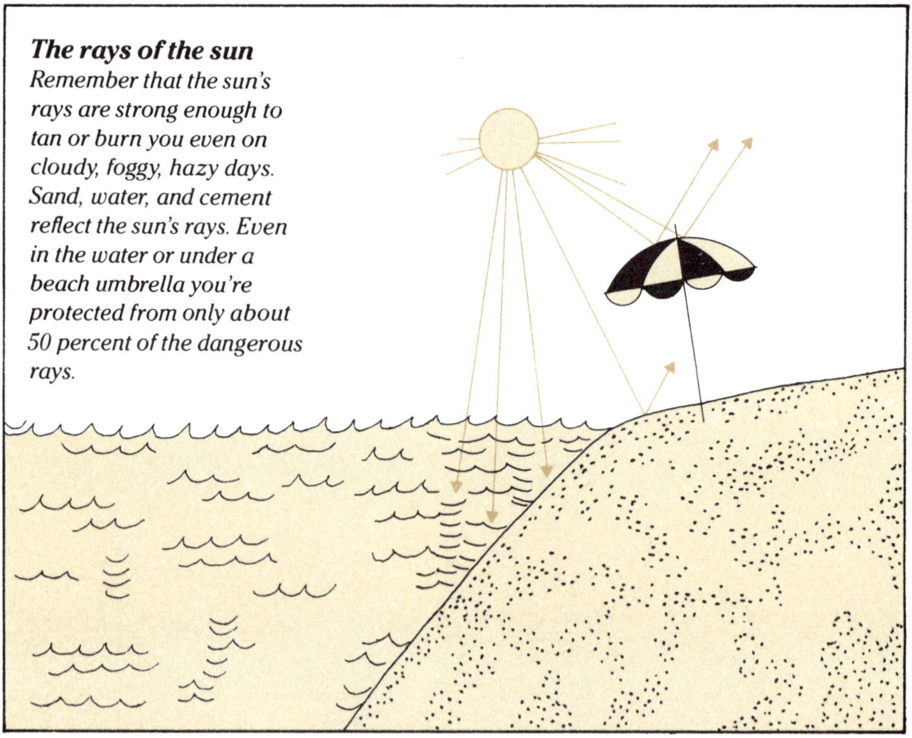

The rays of the sun
Remember that the sun's rays are strong enough to tan or burn you even on cloudy, foggy, hazy days. Sand, water, and cement reflect the sun's rays. Even in the water or under a beach umbrella you're protected from only about 50 percent of the dangerous rays.

Melanin

Skin contains melanin, the pigment that determines our skin color. Melanin also protects the skin by absorbing the sun's dangerous ultraviolet rays. To prevent further damage to our skin, our melanin darkens as we're exposed to the sun's cancer-causing radiation.

Basking in the sun isn't as dangerous for dark-

Sunscreen tips
Use your sunscreen on all exposed areas of skin. Apply it a few minutes before going out into the sunlight so that your skin can absorb it.

skinned people as it is for light-skinned people. Though dark-skinned people can burn, the development of skin cancer among them is fairly rare—but skin damage that results in premature aging happens. However, among light-skinned people, it's easy to burn and damage the skin. Light-skinned people are most likely to wrinkle and develop skin cancer—in fact, light-skinned people are 5 times more likely to develop skin cancer than are dark-skinned people.

Skin cancer is the most common form of cancer, and the chief cause of skin cancer is exposure to the sun. Because of this, skin cancer is most common on areas of the body exposed to the sun and is more common in rural populations—people who work outdoors—than in city populations.

The cause of sunburn is exposure to ultraviolet light. What actually happens when you "cook" your skin in the sun is that it turns red and painful just as if you had put your body into an oven. The redness is caused by additional blood flow to the area—your body is trying to heal itself.

As exposure to the sun continues, your skin will turn darker because of the damage being done—your skin is using its melanin to prevent further damage. Your tan is the result of the immediate damage done to your skin by the sun. However, long-range damage is also being done to your skin. Even your tan can't protect you against the damaging effects of sun exposure.

From underneath the skin, your body attempts to repair the damage already done by sending new skin cells up to replace the burned cells; your old cells are being shed faster than normally, and this causes the peeling associated with sunburn.

Treatment for sunburn

You'll need to soothe the pain of your sunburn while the skin repairs itself.

1. Apply an ointment containing a local anesthetic, such as first-aid ointments, or specific sunburn sprays or creams. Products containing PABA (Para-Aminobenzoic Acid) help relieve the discomfort of sunburn.

2. Use cool compresses of witch hazel; or Burow's solution (1 tablespoon to 1 quart water); or baking soda (3 tablespoons to 1 quart of water); or Domeboro or Blueboro powder (according to directions on the package). Apply compresses for about 15 minutes several times a day.

Black skin needs protection, too
It's not true that black skin needs no protection. Although black skin is far less likely to burn than white skin, it'll age prematurely if subjected to long-term exposure.

3. Cool baths and showers help to reduce pain and may also prevent or limit the amount of blistering.

4. Keep your skin well moisturized while it's healing.

5. Take aspirin to relieve the swelling, redness, and pain. If you can't take aspirin, an aspirin substitute will also reduce discomfort.

6. Drink plenty of fluids to replenish those lost through perspiration and dehydration.

7. If these steps have not greatly improved your condition in 2 to 3 days, see a doctor. You may need a prescription cream of hydrocortisone or hydrocortisone in oral or injection form.

Prevention of sunburn

Regardless of your skin type, protect yourself when outdoors by using sunscreens—creams, lotions, and makeup that screen out the sun's harmful rays.

A wide variety of these products is available, and they've been rated as to their SPF (Sun Protection Factor). The SPF ranges from 2 to 15 according to the degree to which the product blocks out the sun's radiation. The higher the SPF, the more effective the product is in preventing sunburn.

PABA is frequently used in sunscreens and sun lotions. It's preferable to use a product containing PABA because PABA filters out undesirable ultraviolet B rays, which do much damage and contribute to skin cancer. PABA allows ultraviolet A rays to penetrate so that you can tan if you wish but at a slower, safer rate. Some skins are sensitive to both A and B type rays and must be protected by a product rated 15.

Skin types and recommended SPF

This chart matches skin types to recommended SPF ratings. Find your skin type in the column at left and read across to find the recommended SPF.

Skin type	Recommended SPF
Burns easily; never tans	8 or higher
Burns easily; tans minimally	6 to 7
Burns moderately; tans gradually	4 to 5
Rarely burns; always tans well	2 to 3
Rarely burns; tans easily	2

Choose the right sunscreen and use it correctly

Know your skin type and be aware of how much sun exposure you can tolerate without becoming burned.

Sunscreens must be reapplied periodically. Perspiring and swimming will wash off sunscreens. Always dry your skin thoroughly when you come out of the water—drops of water act like little mirrors and intensify the sun's burning effect.

Some sunscreen products are advertised as "waterproof." However, with these the protection is lost if you remain in the water for more than 30 minutes. The "waterproof" lotions shouldn't be dried off. If you use one, let the air dry your skin.

If you must be outdoors between 10 and 2, use a sunscreen with a higher rating or reduce the length of your exposure.

Relief from sunburn pain

Sunscreens and lotions containing PABA help relieve the discomfort of a sunburn. However, sunscreens that don't contain PABA won't relieve sunburn pain and may irritate damaged skin.

Remember that the sun's rays are strong enough to tan or burn even on cloudy, foggy, hazy days. Sand, water, and cement (such as that around swimming pools) reflect the sun's rays. Even under a beach umbrella, you're only protected from about 50 percent of the dangerous rays.

Avoid exposure during the most dangerous hours—when the sun is directly overhead. This is usually between 10 A.M. and 2 P.M. Early morning (before 10) and late afternoon (after 4) are the safest times of the day for enjoying the beach, pool, or outdoor activities.

If you become burned, stay out of the sun and let your skin heal. Remember that after your skin has peeled, you're once again just as vulnerable to burning as you were before the first burn.

Never try to acquire or maintain a tan at a "tanning salon." No matter what assurances of protection they offer, you're risking wrinkles, premature aging, and skin cancer by exposure to radiation from ultraviolet lamps.

Sun poisoning

Sunburn is a form of sun poisoning. However, there are other symptoms that occur as a reaction to exposure to the sun. These include itch, rash, blisters, and an intensified sunburn. This intensified sunburn is out of all proportion to the degree of exposure and previous experience with your skin's tolerance to sunlight. This reaction is called photosensitivity (sensitivity to light). It may also trigger virus-related disorders of the skin such as herpes simplex (cold sores) and lupus (inflammatory dermatitis).

The term *sun poisoning* refers to an adverse physical reaction, a "sun allergy," caused by sun exposure in combination with other substances. People with a poor supply of melanin are especially vulnerable.

Causes of sun poisoning

Among the substances known to cause the allergic type of reaction known as sun poisoning are:

- Medications taken orally, including antibiotics such as tetracycline and sulfa drugs, diabetes medication, high blood pressure medication, certain drugs given for fungus infections, and a variety of tranquilizers.

- Certain substances found in cosmetics, soaps, shampoos, and even suntan lotions, such as the antiseptic bithionol.

Prescription drugs and photosensitivity

Some prescription drugs may cause what's called a photosensitivity reaction in your skin when you go out in the sun. The skin may redden worse than with a sunburn, blister, and peel, or you may get an allergic reaction, like a rash. Sunscreens aren't always reliable in preventing a photosensitive reaction, although they do provide some protection. Be especially cautious if you're taking oral antibiotics such as democycline, doxycycline, or tetracycline. Large doses of Vitamin A, sometimes prescribed for acne, are also a photosensitizer, as is the tranquilizer chlorpromazine. Check with your doctor if you're taking a prescription drug and you're not sure about its effects.

- Various plants, fruits, and vegetables—particularly carrots, celery, parsnips, and limes—coming into contact with your skin while you're exposed to the sun.

Treatment for sun poisoning

1. Apply wet compresses soaked in baking soda solution, Burow's solution, Domeboro powder, or Blueboro powder.

2. Take soothing baths using specially prepared oils for treating dry skin.

3. Certain nonprescription sleep aids contain antihistamines and can provide restful and comfortable nights; take an antihistamine if the itching is very troublesome.

4. Smooth a moisturizing cream or lotion on your skin.

5. Drink plenty of fluids.

6. See a doctor if your symptoms persist or get worse.

Prevention of sun poisoning

1. Use the trial-and-error method of discovering which substance or substances trigger your allergic reaction.

2. If the problem is caused by a medication that would be dangerous or life-threatening to eliminate, you'll have to avoid exposure to the sun.

3. Always use a sunscreen when exposed to the sun's rays.

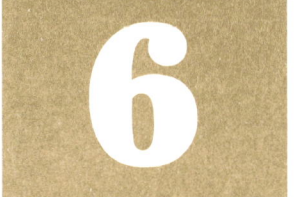

Allergy-related disorders

An allergy is your body's overreaction or sensitivity to a particular substance. Allergy-producing substances, or allergens, are all around us—in the air we breathe, in our food and drink, in the clothes we wear, and in the things we touch.

There's no rhyme or reason to allergic reactions. Seemingly innocent substances can trigger violent reactions in certain people. For example, only one member of a large family may be sensitive to a certain food. Or two family members may develop the same allergy—one in infancy and the other in middle age. However, most people with allergies develop them early in life. Some people never suffer from allergies; others develop numerous allergies.

Sometimes a substance with which you have come into contact for years—with no adverse reaction—will suddenly trigger an allergic reaction.

Some allergies cause symptoms in your nose and other parts of your respiratory system (running nose or wheezing, for example); other allergies cause symptoms in your intestinal tract (such as nausea or diarrhea).

Allergens usually affect the part of the body they contact, but it's not unusual for an allergic reaction to cause symptoms in other locations. For example, an allergen that you eat may react on your skin—you might eat strawberries and break out in hives. An inhaled allergen might cause you to develop a rash.

Contact dermatitis
Contact dermatitis may appear when the skin comes into contact with an allergen. The symptoms of contact dermatitis include inflammation, redness, itching, swelling, blisters, and welts. There may also be intestinal problems, respiratory problems, and neurological problems (such as migraine headaches).

Causes of allergic skin reactions
The allergens that cause these symptoms are numerous and varied—almost anything can be the culprit. After much observation, specialists have broken down

---

Allergens
We come in contact with allergens in four ways:
- *They can be inhaled, or breathed in—such as pollen or dust.*
- *They can be ingested, or eaten—such as certain foods.*
- *They can be touched—such as poison ivy.*
- *They can be injected into the body—such as the venom of a bee.*

Insect repellents
Using external insect repellents is a good way to prevent having to use nonprescription medications for bites and stings, unless you're allergic to them. Insect repellents come in the form of sprays, creams, lotions, sticks, or on towelettes. You should cover all exposed parts of your body with the repellent, avoiding the eyes, lips, and areas with cuts or sunburn. Read the label to make sure the product won't stain clothes. There are no approved ingredients you can take internally to ward off unwelcome insect attackers.

the causes of allergic skin reactions into the following categories:

1. What you wear

Parts of jewelry or clothing containing nickel can cause allergic reactions. Nickel is frequently used in earrings, watches, rings, bracelets, necklaces, zippers, bra hooks, eyeglass frames, snaps, and hairpins. Approximately 11 percent of people wearing articles containing nickel develop an allergy to it.

Clothing may contain a substance to which you are sensitive. The allergic reaction will occur on the skin area that comes in contact with the clothing.

Clothing made from leather, such as shoes, pocketbooks, wallets, gloves, hatbands, jackets, pants, and skirts, may contain the chemical potassium dichromate, commonly used in tanning leather. About 8 percent of people are allergic to this substance.

Some people experience allergic reactions to the adhesives, chemicals, or rubber compounds used in some clothing and shoes.

Wool, fur, silk, elastic, and certain synthetic fibers are common allergens.

The chemicals used in "permanent press" or "anti-shrink" garments can trigger allergic reactions. The same is true of some fabric softeners.

Formaldehyde, used in "wash-and-wear" fabrics, cotton, and rayon, is another common allergen.

Any fabric—not only in clothing but also in upholstery, towels, bed linens—that has been prepared with dyes may cause a reaction. Black, dark blue, and dark brown are the most common offenders.

2. What you touch around the house

Antiseptics, found in many household cleaning products, can cause allergic reactions. Ten percent of users are allergic to the ingredient thimerosal; 8 percent are allergic to merthiolate.

Common sources of hand dermatitis—also known as housewives' eczema—are bleaches, waxes, detergents, polishes, cleansers, soaps, and fabric softeners.

Frequent contact with the juices of certain vegetables (particularly potatoes, tomatoes, garlic); certain fruits (particularly oranges and grapefruits); and various spices can irritate the skin and cause an allergic reaction.

Various houseplants (particularly the bulb variety, such as hyacinth and tulip) cause skin reactions.

3. What you put on your skin

Other allergy sources
You may be allergic to a product worn by someone else with whom you are in close contact, such as your hairdresser or barber.

Nonprescription preparations, such as insect repellants; toilet paper; hemorrhoid creams; liniments; medicated creams and lotions for acne, athlete's foot, and eczema; and remedies for poison ivy all contain chemicals (such as benzocaine and zirconium) that may cause an allergic reaction.

4. What you touch outdoors

Pesticides, fertilizers, and insecticides contain known allergens.

Trees, such as elm, white pine, citrus, Norway spruce; flowers, such as asters, daffodils, sunflowers, lilies, lilacs; weeds and grasses, such as ragweed, gold-

Cosmetics and allergic reactions

Cosmetics may cause allergic reactions. Any of the thousands of products we use on our skin and hair can cause allergic reactions in sensitive people. Among the products that may cause an allergic reaction are:

aftershave lotion	eyeliner	mask
antiperspirant	eyeshadow	moisturizer
artificial nails	face cream	nail base coat
astringent	false eyelashes	nail conditioner
bath oil	glue for eyelashes	nail hardener
bath salts	glue for hairpieces	nail polish
bleach	glue for nails	nail top coat
blusher	hand cream	perfume
body lotion	hair color	powder
bubble bath	hair spray	setting lotion
cleansers	hair straightener	shampoo
cologne	hair tonic	shaving cream
cream rinse	lip gloss	soap
cuticle remover	lip liner	sun lotion
deodorant	lipstick	sunscreen
depilatory	lotion	toner
douche	makeup base	topical anesthetic
eyebrow pencil	mascara	

All of these products contain a variety of natural and chemical substances, any one of which may cause an allergic reaction. You can never be certain you're allergy-free. Sometimes, a product that has never caused an adverse reaction will suddenly "turn" on you. This is because you can develop a sensitivity after long exposure. Furthermore, the manufacturer may change the formula for a product, exposing you to a new substance.

Three plants to avoid

These three related plants deserve special attention. All three produce an oil, called urushiol, that is a potent allergen. Urushiol is most abundant in the leaves and stems of these plants, but it's present in all parts, and contact with any part of the plant can cause a reaction. You can develop a poison ivy reaction in any season—even during the winter, when the plants are dried up, the urushiol is present.

Some people develop dermatitis from minute particles carried through the air in the smoke of burning brush that contains one of these plants. The urushiol can also be spread by anything that comes in contact with it—pets, sports equipment, gardening tools. Thus, you don't need to touch a plant to come in contact with the urushiol—petting a dog or picking up a golf club can bring you in contact with the allergen.

Poison ivy

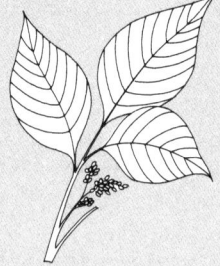

- Leaves always consist of three glossy leaflets
- Grows as a small plant, a vine, or a shrub
- Grows everywhere in the United States except California and parts of adjacent states

Poison oak

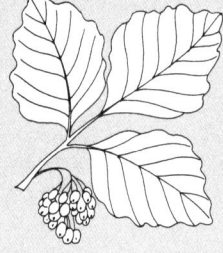

- Leaves always consist of three leaflets
- Grows as a shrub or vine
- Grows in California and parts of adjacent states

Poison sumac

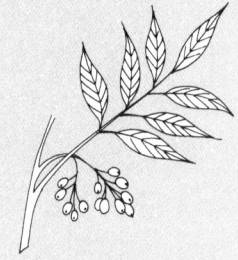

- Grows as a woody shrub or small tree from 5 to 25 feet tall
- Grows in most of the eastern third of the United States

enrod, clover, crabgrass; vegetables, such as asparagus, garlic, parsnips, turnips; and thousands of other growing things can cause contact dermatitis.

Poison ivy, poison oak, and poison sumac
These three related plants deserve special attention. All three produce an oil, called urushiol, that is a potent allergen. Urushiol is most abundant in the leaves and stems of these plants, but it's present in all parts, and contact with any part of the plant can cause a re-

You may be susceptible
Even if you've never had a bad reaction to poison ivy, oak, or sumac, you may become susceptible. For some people, it takes many years of repeated exposures to develop a sensitivity. Some people never develop the allergy; some are allergic all their lives.

action. You can develop a poison ivy reaction in any season—even during the winter, when the plants are dried up, the urushiol is present.

Some people develop dermatitis from minute particles carried through the air in the smoke of burning brush that contains one of these plants. The urushiol can also be spread by anything that comes in contact with it—pets, sports equipment, gardening tools. Thus, you don't need to touch a plant to come in contact with the urushiol—petting a dog or picking up a golf club can bring you in contact with the allergen.

Symptoms of poison ivy, oak, or sumac dermatitis

After contact with one of these plants, the first symptoms of itching and burning may appear in a matter of hours but usually develop within 24 to 48 hours in a sensitized person. The skin that has touched the plant or the urushiol becomes red, then bumps and watery blisters appear. There is also usually itching and swelling. The rash reaches its worst after about 5 days and then gradually improves within a week or two even without treatment. The blisters break, and the oozing sores begin to crust over and disappear.

Treatment for poison ivy, oak, or sumac dermatitis

1. The first and most essential part of treatment is to immediately wash the affected area with soap and cold water. Use yellow laundry soap or Fels Naptha if available and lather several times, rinsing the area in running water after each sudsing.

2. You can relieve the itching and burning by applying compresses soaked in cold water or Burow's solution. Calamine lotion spread over the rash will help relieve the itching and burning and will also help keep the area dry.

3. Baths in which Domeboro or Blueboro powder has been dissolved can help alleviate your discomfort. If the affected area isn't large, apply wet compresses using one of these powder solutions.

4. For more severe cases with widespread rash and itch, you'll need drugs such as an antihistamine or a corticosteroid. If your rash becomes infected, you'll also need an antibiotic.

Occupational contact dermatitis

Are you allergic to allergens in your workplace? Ten

Skin tests for allergies
If your doctor suspects you're having an allergic reaction to a cosmetic or another substance, he may give you a skin test to determine the cause of your reaction.

Your doctor will use an allergen extract in one of three tests. In a scratch test, he'll scrape the surface of your skin and apply the extract. In a prick test, he'll apply the extract to your arm and then prick your skin. With the intradermal test, he'll inject the extract just under the surface of the skin.

If you've swelling or redness after one of these tests, you may have an allergy to the substance in the extract.

Don't try to interpret your own test. Only your doctor can judge your reaction correctly.

percent of all skin disorders in the United States are job-related. Fortunately, 80 percent of occupational contact dermatitis affects only the hands. This is because the allergy-causing substances are handled.

In more than 55,000 occupations, people are exposed to potential allergens. Sometimes the allergic reaction appears almost immediately, but in many cases it may take more than 50 years for the allergy to develop.

Treatment for contact dermatitis

1. Determine the cause of the reaction and either eliminate it or avoid it. If you can't avoid it entirely, try switching products or changing your habits. You and your doctor should join forces in detecting the substance that is causing your reaction.

2. To relieve the symptoms, follow these steps:

• Take lukewarm baths using Burow's solution, Epsom salts, Domeboro or Blueboro powder.

• Use cool, wet compresses soaked in one of the above.

• Avoid extreme heat or cold temperatures—these aggravate an itch.

• Apply soothing creams to avoid dryness of the skin.

• Soap has a drying effect on skin—use soap substitutes and avoid excessive washing and drying.

• To relieve the itching, take a nonprescription antihistamine.

• Switch to hypoallergenic products.

• Avoid all perfumes and perfumed products.

• Don't wear rubber gloves. These are a frequent cause of allergic reactions. Use glove liners or try plastic gloves instead if you're trying to avoid hand contact with a substance.

• Wear protective clothing when outdoors.

• If you come in contact with something to which you're allergic, cleanse the area thoroughly as soon as possible.

If your symptoms persist or get worse:

1. Make sure you have identified the actual allergen and avoid it.

2. Use nonprescription products such as mild cortisone creams.

Identifying the offender

When trying to identify the substance causing the allergic reaction, don't rule out a cosmetic or laundry product—even if you've been using the product for many years without experiencing any reaction. Manufacturers sometimes change the formula for a cosmetic or laundry product without informing consumers, some of whom may then become allergic to a previously harmless product.

Job-related skin disorders

Many people come in contact with allergens at work. The following chart matches occupations with some possible allergy-causing substances:

Occupation	Possible allergens
Auto mechanic	Paints, lacquer, grease, solvents, oils, cleansers, rubber, cement, chrome
Butcher	Animal hairs, meat, insecticides
Clothing worker	Wool, fur, feathers, dyes, benzene, turpentine
Dry cleaner	Carbon tetrachloride, benzene, turpentine
Exterminator	Arsenic, formaldehyde, chemical insecticides
Farmer, mail carrier, outdoor worker	Insect stings, animal bites, insecticides, extreme weather conditions, trees, plants (including grasses and poison ivy)
Florist and landscape gardener	Chrysanthemums, ivy, geraniums, tulips, molds, fungi, fertilizers, pesticides
Hairdresser and barber	Shampoos, dyes, bleaches
Homemaker and domestic worker	Bleaches, disinfectants, insecticides, detergents, polishes
Jeweler	Nickel, chrome, solvents, jewelers' rouge
Medical personnel	Antibiotics, rubber, plastic, anesthetics, antiseptics, disinfectants
Office worker	Typewriter ribbons, carbon paper, nickel, glue, ink
Painter	Turpentine, lead, dyes, solvents, oils, thinners, paints
Poultry dealer	Feathers, mites, insects

Honeybee

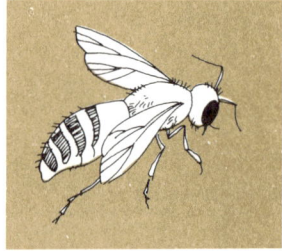

Honeybees have round, smooth abdomens and build nests in hollow trees or in the ground. They can be quite aggressive when defending the area around their nests. They release "alarm odors" that alert other nearby bees to join in the attack on a victim, and this can lead to multiple stings.

Bumblebee

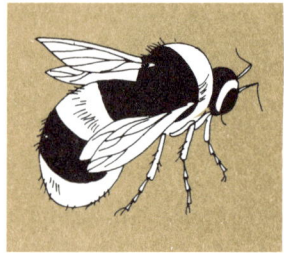

Bumblebees are 2 to 3 times larger than honeybees, have furry, rounded abdomens, and make a noisy buzzing sound. They aren't as aggressive as honeybees and will rarely attack unless a nest, located in the ground, is stepped upon.

3. See your doctor. He or she will probably prescribe a cortisone-type cream to relieve inflammation and perhaps a medicated cream to combat dryness.

4. If your case is very severe, your doctor will probably give you pills of the cortisone-steroid variety and a prescription antihistamine. If an infection has developed, you'll need an antibiotic.

Insect stings

As efficient as the skin is at protecting us from foreign invaders in the form of bacteria and harmful substances, it's not impenetrable. Insect stings can break through the skin.

Most insect stings are only uncomfortable or slightly painful. However, they can be dangerous; occasionally, they're fatal. A first sting won't result in a strong reaction; sensitivity must be built up. If you experience a very severe reaction to an insect sting, you've already been sensitized by a previous sting. Consult your doctor if you have reason to believe that you're highly sensitive to insect stings. It may be advisable for you to undergo desensitization, a series of injections made up of extracts of insect venom. This treatment will immunize you against possible violent reactions in the future.

Only a very small percentage of the population is highly allergic to insect stings. An allergic person's reaction to an insect sting can be severe and, in extreme cases, can lead to death in a very short time. If you or someone you're with experiences an excessive reaction to a sting—particularly if the victim is having breathing difficulties—immediate emergency medical help is essential.

Wasps, hornets, bees, and yellow jackets are the insects most often associated with stings. Many people confuse bees and yellow jackets, but their stings differ in one very important way: when a bee stings, it embeds its stinger in your skin. When the bee tries to free itself, its stinger breaks off (injured in this way the bee soon dies). The stinger remains stuck in your skin; attached to the stinger is a venom sac, which continues pumping venom into your skin for a short period. The stinger and attached venom sac must be removed, but don't use tweezers. Squeezing the stinger will only pump more venom into your body; instead, scrape the stinger away with a fingernail or the blade of a knife.

Hornet

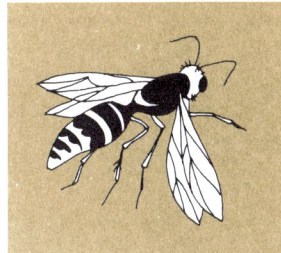

Hornets hang their large, pear-shaped nests from tree limbs. They don't attack unless their nest is threatened.

Yellow jacket

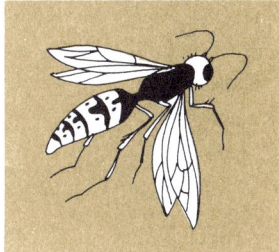

Yellow jackets build their nests in trees, holes in the ground, tree stumps, or walls. They're very aggressive and quick-tempered.

Symptoms of insect stings

Following the pinprick of the sting (which may not be noticed), you'll have pain, swelling, redness, and itching at the site of the sting.

Treatment for insect stings

1. If you've been stung by a bee, you'll have to remove the stinger. Remember not to use tweezers.

2. Cleanse the area around the sting with soap and water.

3. Apply a paste of meat tenderizer and water (one quarter of a teaspoon of tenderizer added to about one or two teaspoons of water) to the sting. This will stop the pain.

4. Apply calamine lotion or a specially medicated nonprescription cream or lotion every 4 hours to relieve the itching.

5. If there's a great deal of swelling, take an antihistamine.

6. If possible, keep the affected area above the heart.

7. Applying an ice cube to an insect sting for several minutes will reduce the swelling and relieve the itching.

8. If your symptoms persist or worsen, see a doctor. You may need an injection of antihistamine or a corticosteroid drug.

Prevention of insect stings

To avoid insect stings, stay away from wasps, hornets, bees, and yellow jackets. If you spot one nearby, don't overreact. Just walk away. In addition, take these precautions:

• Don't wear perfume or any sweet-smelling product outdoors. Insects will mistake you for a flower.

• Don't go near hives or nests.

• Apply insect repellent to your exposed skin and clothing when outdoors.

• Remember that bright, light-colored clothes attract insects.

• Don't go barefoot around bees or other insects.

• When eating outside, keep sweet foods and beverages covered.

• If you know you're sensitive, carry an anti-sting emergency kit. Available only with a doctor's prescription, each kit contains antihistamine tablets, alcohol swabs, and a preloaded syringe filled with epinephrine.

If you feel uneasy about injecting yourself, an automatic injector called EpiPen is available, also by prescription only. All you have to do is release the safety cap and press the device to your thigh. Of course, if you've already suffered bad reactions to insect stings, you should ask your doctor about immunization.

Hives
Rather than a disease, hives is a symptom of a disorder within your body. Although usually the result of an allergy, hives can also be caused by an infection or emotional stress.

Removing a stinger

Bees have barbed stingers that become firmly anchored in human skin. When the bee tries to free itself—or when the victim brushes it off—the stinger and its attached venom sac break off. Minus this part of its body, the bee flies off and dies; the stinger, embedded in the skin, continues to pump venom into the victim.

If you're stung by a bee, you'll need to remove the bee's stinger before performing any other first-aid measures. Don't use tweezers to remove a stinger. Squeezing the stinger will only release more venom into the wound. Scrape away the stinger with a fingernail or the edge of a knife blade. Having removed the stinger, wash the wound with soap and water and apply an antiseptic. If available, apply ice to the wound. This will help reduce the swelling.

The pain and irritation can be relieved with the application of a paste made from baking soda and water; however, some doctors recommend the application of meat tenderizer (any brand will do). Make a paste of ¹/₄ of a teaspoon of meat tenderizer added to about 1 or 2 teaspoons of water.

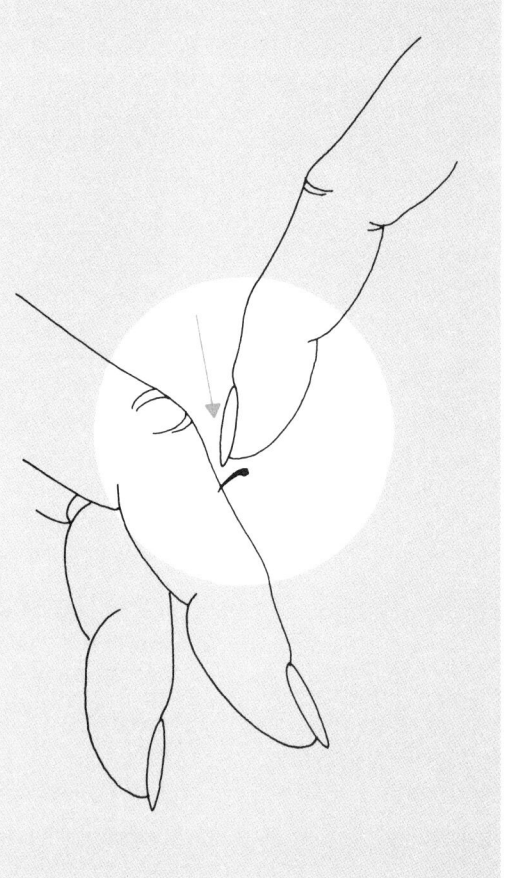

Anti-sting emergency kit

If you know you're sensitive, carry an anti-sting emergency kit. Available only with a doctor's prescription, each kit contains antihistamine tablets, alcohol swabs, and a preloaded syringe filled with epinephrine. If you feel uneasy about injecting yourself, an automatic injector called EpiPen is available, also by prescription only. All you have to do is release the safety cap and press the device to your thigh. Of course, if you've already suffered bad reactions to insect stings, you should ask your doctor about immunization.

Most common culprits

The most common hives-causing foods are strawberries, oranges, bananas, milk, eggs, nuts, and seafood. The most common drugs are penicillin and aspirin; food preservatives are other frequent culprits. Common airborne offenders include dust, mold, pollen, and animal dander.

Be a detective

Chronic or recurrent cases of hives demand good detective work. In addition to skin testing for common allergens, you may need a thorough physical evaluation and sophisticated blood and lab tests.

Allergy-caused hives usually follow an insect sting, eating a particular food, taking a particular drug, or contact with a fabric or product to which you've become sensitive. However, almost anything can produce an eruption of hives.

Symptoms of hives

The most common symptoms of hives are welts or swellings of various sizes and shapes surrounded by reddened skin. This swelling is accompanied by itching, burning, or stinging. Hives also resemble blisters and may be filled with a yellowish fluid.

The legs, thighs, buttocks, and back of the neck are the most frequent locations for hives. However, huge, disfiguring hives may erupt on the face, particularly the lips and eyelids. On occasion, hives may affect the throat, swelling so severely that emergency medical treatment is needed to prevent suffocation.

Treatment for hives

1. Relieve the itching and other uncomfortable symptoms with lukewarm or cool baths. Don't use soap (which is drying to the skin) but, rather, soothing bath oils.

2. Apply medicated creams, ointments, lotions—particularly calamine lotion—every 4 hours.

3. Take a nonprescription antihistamine.

4. Avoid wearing too many clothes or taking part in activities that make you excessively warm, for perspiration aggravates hives.

5. If your hives persist or become worse, see your doctor. Very likely, he or she will give you an injection of an antibiotic, a corticosteroid medication, or prescription cream.

6. Try to determine the cause of your hives. This may not be easy—the possible causes are almost limitless. However, the most common hives-causing foods, drugs, and airborne substances are known. You can be tested for these by your doctor, and after identifying the substance responsible, you can try to avoid it.

7. With a sudden outbreak of hives, you can narrow the probable causes more easily. Did you eat something you've never eaten before? Did you just start taking a drug? Were you exposed to some unusual animal or plant? Were you emotionally upset?

7

Virus-related disorders

Cold sores

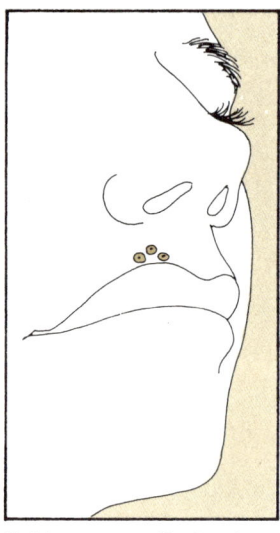

Cold sores usually develop on your lips or around your mouth. You may have a small cluster of tiny blisters.

Cold sores and dental work
A visit to the dentist can lead to cold sores. The pulling and pushing of the skin inside the mouth and the dryness caused by dental operations can cause the irritation necessary for cold sores.

A virus is a living organism smaller than bacteria. Viruses are responsible for many different diseases, often called viral infections. Viral infections can't be cured but must "run their course." However, steps can be taken to relieve the symptoms of viral infections.

Cold sores, fever blisters, herpes simplex

Cold sores, also called fever blisters, are recurrent viral infections caused by herpes simplex. This disorder is common, unattractive, and uncomfortable. It's also highly contagious and difficult to treat. Fortunately, it's rarely dangerous.

Causes of cold sores

The herpes simplex virus is responsible for cold sores. This virus may remain dormant in your body for many years. In fact, you may never develop a cold sore. Some people seem to be prone to them and suffer recurrent outbreaks. Usually, the first episode of infection occurs in childhood.

Factors that trigger an eruption include:

• Colds (hence the names "cold sores" and "fever blisters")

• Exposure to the sun

• Emotional stress

• Certain foods, particularly common allergens such as chocolate, shellfish, and peanuts

• Menstruation

• Damage to the skin, such as that incurred from pulling and stretching of your mouth and lips during dentistry

Symptoms of cold sores

Cold sores usually develop on your lips or around your mouth. However, they can occur on any part of your body.

• The first symptom is a tiny reddened area that is somewhat painful. Within approximately 8 hours a

The infection may spread
In rare cases, the herpes simplex infection may spread, causing a secondary infection in another body organ or eyesight-damaging lesions on the cornea of the eye.

small cluster of tiny blisters may form around it. The blisters—or single blister—are raised and filled with watery fluid. The size varies from that of a pinhead to over a half-inch in diameter.

- Cold sore blisters are painful but may also itch, burn, or tingle.
- After a week or 10 days, healing begins. During this time, the blisters become yellow and crusty and finally form scabs that are still somewhat painful.
- Healing is usually complete in 2 weeks, but occasionally the infection spreads, causing swelling of the lymph glands in your neck, and is accompanied by pain.

Treatment for cold sores
Because cold sores will heal themselves, treatment consists of relieving the discomforts that accompany them:

1. Apply a cold compress or ice cube.
2. Take aspirin or an aspirin substitute to relieve pain and reduce possible fever.
3. Certain nonprescription "cold sore" products, such as Campho-Phenique or Blistex, can help soothe the discomfort.
4. Avoid acidic foods, especially citrus juices and fruits. Eat soft and alkaline foods such as bananas and vegetables.
5. If you develop cold sores frequently, apply tincture of benzoin or Vaseline between episodes to keep your skin in the susceptible area from developing cracks or becoming irritated.
6. Before going out in the sun, apply a sunscreen to your lips, such as number 15 sunscreen, or zinc oxide.
7. If your symptoms persist or recur often, see your doctor. You may require a prescribed oral antibiotic.

Shingles
Shingles, the proper name of which is herpes zoster, affects 1 million Americans each year. It's caused by the same virus that's responsible for chicken pox, but shingles is far more severe than either chicken pox or its relative, herpes simplex (cold sores).

Zoster
The name zoster is derived from a Greek word meaning "belt."

Like chicken pox, shingles usually occurs only once in a lifetime. However, shingles occasionally recurs twice or three times and affects the same or different parts of the body. Shingles is only mildly contagious.

The shingles and chicken pox virus remains in your body throughout your life. Most children contract chicken pox. After this occurs, an immunity to this virus may be established, and the virus remains dormant for many years. In fact, it may never erupt again.

However, as people grow older—from about age 30 on—the immunity developed early in life wears off. At this point, the virus can erupt and multiply. About 20 percent of adults are afflicted with shingles at some time. Although the disease may occur at any age, it's far more apt to strike older people. Individuals in their seventies are 15 times more prone to shingles than are youngsters.

Even so, children or young people may get shingles if they never had chicken pox or if they had it but didn't develop an immunity to the virus. Periods of immunity vary from person to person. Some people are never immune; others are never susceptible. This depends on each person's immune system.

Shingles is a herpes infection of a nerve in the brain or spinal cord. The infection travels a specific nerve route, setting up inflammation—crops of small blisters—and pain. The virus will attack one of any peripheral (body surface) nerves. It then follows along the pathway of this nerve.

The nerves affected are usually those from the middle of the back around one side of the body to the navel. Shingles usually occurs on only one side and is comparable to half a belt. Because of the pain and misery associated with shingles, the Norwegians have given the disease an apt name: "a belt of roses from Hell."

Shingles may affect any body area, including the face, scalp, arms, hands, or legs.

Causes of shingles

Lowered resistance because of physical or emotional stress can make you susceptible to an outbreak of shingles. You may have heard it said that shingles is a result of "nerves"; this is somewhat true. Stressful periods can create a chemical disturbance in the victim, and the shingles virus may take advantage of this disturbance and erupt.

- A recent illness of another kind may decrease a person's natural immunity.

- An injury that in some way traumatizes a nerve may tend to provoke the disorder.

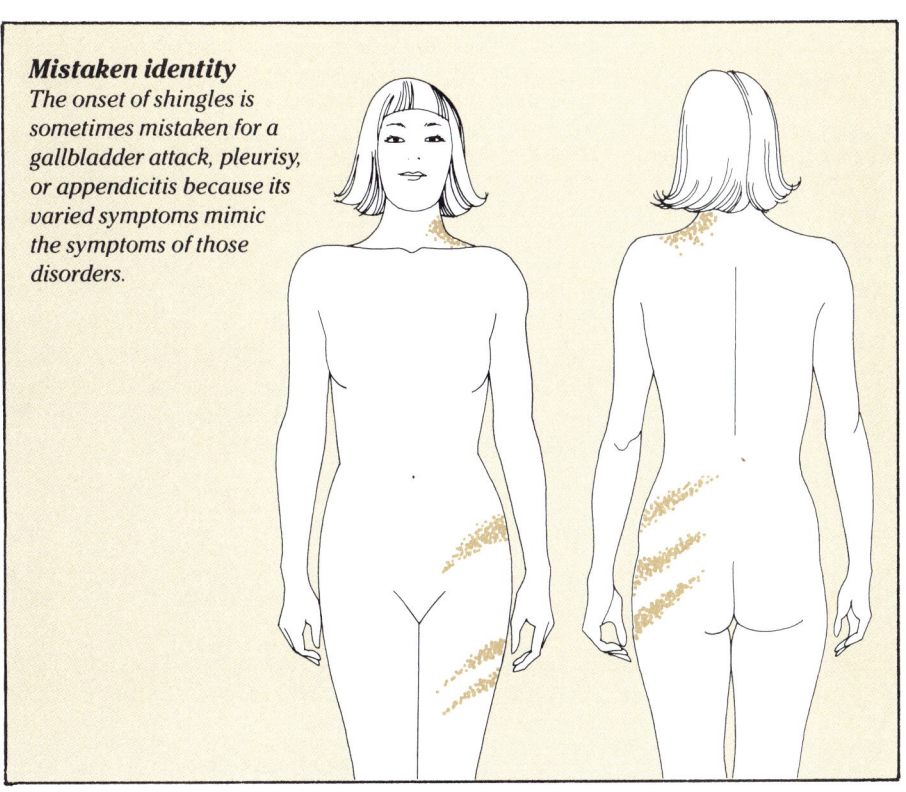

Mistaken identity
The onset of shingles is sometimes mistaken for a gallbladder attack, pleurisy, or appendicitis because its varied symptoms mimic the symptoms of those disorders.

- Immunosuppression—the lowering of the body's natural immune system—may leave the body open to attack by shingles. Drugs that suppress the immune system are frequently used in the treatment of cancer or to help the body accept an organ transplant. These drugs leave a patient open to infections of all kinds, including shingles.

Symptoms of shingles

Early symptoms of shingles appear 3 to 4 days before the rash appears and include a "sick" feeling, fatigue, headache, slight fever, chills, with or without mild to sharp pain in the affected area. There may also be localized itching, burning, or "drawing" sensations. The discomforts may be steady or intermittent (such as sudden sharp jabs of pain).

A reddish rash then appears and soon turns into blisters. These blisters may be small or as large as a 25-cent coin. Filling with fluid, these blisters become firmer and firmer until, after 5 to 7 days, they burst, leaving poxlike sores in the affected area.

Scabs and crusts gradually form and remain for 2 to 5 weeks before the last one falls off.

- Because shingles is a systemic (involving the entire body) infection, it is accompanied by such symptoms as fatigue, fever, and a general sick feeling.

- The pain of shingles is limited to the affected area but may be moderate to agonizing. The inflammation may be light or may involve a thick covering of sores. Swelling of the affected area and temporary paralysis of arm, leg, or chest muscles are not uncommon.

- If shingles affect the face, serious complications may arise if the sores form on the cornea of the eye. These may cause permanent damage to vision—even blindness. Shingles on the face require prompt medical supervision.

- Complications arising from shingles may produce very serious problems, among them viral meningitis, which can be permanent or—in very rare cases—fatal.

- The most common aftereffect of shingles is a neuralgic pain (caused by scarring of the damaged nerve) that may linger long after the attack has passed; sometimes months or even years may go by before this pain disappears completely.

- Scars may be left, particularly where the sores were deepest. Scars will also remain if the lesions become infected.

- Severely decreased energy and a generally unwell feeling may remain long after the sores have healed.

Treatment for shingles

Zovirax (trade name for acylovar) is effective in treating shingles. The earlier the drug is taken in a shingles outbreak, the better the results.

Zovirax decreases the intensity of the pain, shortens the period of extreme pain, and heals the sores about a week sooner than they would otherwise heal.

- Aspirin can be used to relieve pain, but a stronger prescription painkiller is usually required.

- Ice packs can also be helpful in relieving pain.

- In those cases in which shingles affects the face and endangers the eyes, the doctor will prescribe an oral cortisone-type drug or cortisone and antibiotic drops to be put into the eye.

- Compresses moistened with Burow's solution, Domeboro or Blueboro powder solutions, applied for

A promising new drug
Excellent results have been reported in studies using a new drug, adenosine phosphate. If given within the first 3 days of a shingles eruption, this drug reduces pain and other symptoms, shortens the period of the outbreak, and also permanently suppresses the responsible virus. This drug has not yet been approved for use in this country.

Helping lesions heal quicker
You can help your lesions heal quicker by keeping them clean and dry. To help absorb excess moisture, wear cotton underpants. Also, try sprinkling a little cornstarch into your underpants. Wash the lesions several times a day with mild, unscented soap and warm water. Pat your skin dry. Be careful not to scratch the sores.

20 minutes, 4 times a day, decrease inflammation, swelling, and pain, soothe the itching, and aid the drying of the blisters.

• When the blisters begin to dry, a nonprescription anti-itch cream may provide relief.

• If the itching is severe, you may need a nonprescription or prescription antihistamine.

• For neuralgic pain that lingers after the sores have healed, your doctor may prescribe a cortisone-type drug and perhaps a tranquilizer, sedative, or antidepressant.

• Vitamin E oil has been found safe and effective, when applied directly, in reducing scarring.

• Your doctor may prescribe an antibiotic to prevent secondary infections.

Genital herpes

"Herpes" is the common name for a viral infection, transmitted by direct contact, that develops in the form of sores on or around the penis, the vagina, and in the area of the anus and cervix.

As many as 20 million Americans have contracted this disease, raising it to epidemic proportions. Herpes is more prevalent than gonorrhea and syphilis combined. More than a half-million new cases occur each year, appearing most often among white, educated, sexually active men and women between the ages of 20 and 45.

The specific responsible virus is herpes simplex virus (HSV), of which there are two types. HSV-1 usually causes cold sores or fever blisters, and HSV-2 usually causes genital herpes.

However, because of the increased acceptance of oral-genital sexual practices, there's the possibility of cross-infection. In such instances, HSV-1 may result in genital sores, and HSV-2 may produce mouth and lip sores.

Some men and women experience mild or brief attacks; others are very ill during an episode of infection. Also, it's possible to have active, contagious herpes viruses without having any symptoms of genital herpes.

Herpes may remain dormant in a person for many years. However, such "carriers" are still infectious and may transmit an active case of the disease to their sexual partners.

Herpes transmission
When a herpes infection is active, it can be transmitted with a kiss. This occurs because the herpes virus, HSV-2, which causes genital herpes, can—through oral sexual activity—infect a sex partner's lips or mouth. The newly infected person can then transmit the active virus by kissing an uninfected individual. In addition, the herpes virus, HSV-1, which is responsible for cold sores, can—through oral sex—infect a sex partner's genital area.

Other symptoms
A first-time attack of herpes may produce other symptoms, including constipation; bladder, urinary, and menstrual problems; and back pain.

Herpes can also appear after the virus has been long dormant and is suddenly activated by sexual relations. In these cases, the last sex partner may not be responsible for the outbreak.

Symptoms of herpes

Most people with active genital herpes have obvious symptoms in their genital or anal areas.

- Signs of infection will appear in a susceptible person within 4 to 7 days of close contact with a partner who has contagious lesions and secretions.

- With a first attack, the symptoms are most severe and may include fever, headache, stiff neck, muscle pain, joint pain, excruciatingly painful urination or intercourse, swollen lymph glands in the neck or groin, sensitivity to light, and a general feeling of fatigue or illness.

- Burning, itching, sensitivity to touch, tingling, numbness in the affected area, feeling of pressure and intermittent pain are symptoms that rarely occur in the first episode of herpes but usually accompany recurrent attacks. These symptoms may serve as a warning of an impending outbreak and are experienced from 2 hours to 2 days before the sores appear. The various signs may not be confined to the genital-anal area but may also affect the face, lower back, or legs.

- During the first attack and during recurrent attacks, clusters of blisters or fluid- or pus-filled sores appear in or around the affected area. These may itch, burn, tingle, or be very painful. In men, the sores are on the penis or around the anus. In women, they appear around the vagina or on the vulva. In addition, women may have sores inside the vagina or on the cervix. Occasionally, eruptions occur on the abdomen, thighs, face, lips, inside the mouth or throat.

Avoid spreading the infection
Because herpes spreads easily, wash your clothes and bed linens separately from those of other family members. If possible, transfer the laundry directly to the dryer. Otherwise, hang the clothing or bed linens in the sun and iron them later. If this is inconvenient, you may want to send the articles to a professional dry cleaner.

- A discharge from the penis or vagina may be present.

- Within 10 days to 2 weeks, the sores will become crusty, then form scabs, and later heal completely. Scars may remain.

Recurrences

Herpes virus tends to "settle" in nerve routes around the area of the sores. The virus then multiplies. Some of these viruses enter the surrounding nerve fibers from where they move to the nerve cell body and remain there permanently. The virus can be reactivated

When is genital herpes contagious?

Genital herpes is contagious in the active stage—in other words, when you have open, draining sores. Keep in mind that after your initial attack, you may have four or more recurrences a year. Be alert for early signs and symptoms that signal an attack, such as itching, redness, or irritation in your genital area; fever; chills; or a tingling or burning sensation in your thighs or buttocks. Keep track of the active attacks and try to figure out what caused them. Emotional stress or exposure to sunlight, for example, may cause an attack.

Emotional help

Discussion of emotional problems with your doctor is important. Many herpes victims need professional counseling. An organization called HELP/ASHA (Box 100, Palo Alto, California 94302), which has many chapters around the country, provides information and psychological support to its members.

by several factors; how or why this occurs isn't fully understood.

At irregular intervals, the disease will recur but in a much milder form, with far fewer sores, and last from 10 to 12 days. A possible explanation for the decreased severity is that the victim may develop a resistance to the virus.

Repetition of infection occurs approximately 5 to 8 times each year, although some people experience repetitions as frequently as every 3 weeks. Other people may be free of another herpes episode for several years.

Aftereffects and complications

• Emotional trauma

Genital herpes isn't just a painful and distressing ordeal while an attack is in progress—it can also involve ongoing emotional trauma. People with herpes often feel they're unlucky victims; they fear they're a source of danger to their spouses or loved ones. And herpes can cause long-term sexual problems with a spouse. Some herpes sufferers may feel reluctant to engage in sexual relationships because of uncertainty about transmitting herpes. Some people experience no warning signs of an impending attack and may unknowingly spread the infection. There is never a guaranteed "safe" time.

Furthermore, herpes sufferers may shrink from explaining their condition to another person. They fear, too, that no one will want to love them.

Because of problems of loneliness, anger, self-pity—and the fact that the disease is incurable—people with herpes are prone to depression. The black humor that surrounds the disease compounds the problem and may cause people with herpes to feel like modern-day lepers. These emotional consequences of the disease have reached crisis proportions, so much so that psychologists refer to them as "herpes syndrome."

• Pregnant women

A pregnant woman with genital herpes can transmit the virus to her baby in the birth canal at the time of delivery. The baby can acquire a major or even fatal illness. To avoid these potentially devastating consequences, the doctor of a woman with active herpes or a history of herpes may recommend delivery by cesarean section.

- Cancer

Another problem faced by women with herpes is their increased likelihood of developing cancer of the cervix. These women should have a Pap smear test at least once a year in order to detect cancer.

- Herpes keratitis

If the herpes virus is transmitted to the eye from an active sore, a recurrent condition called herpes keratitis may develop. Its symptoms are irritation and pain in the eye and sensitivity to light. This disease requires prompt and continuing medical treatment and supervision, or blindness may result.

Treatment for herpes

Genital herpes can't be cured, but it can be treated. Once the herpes virus gets into the cells, it multiplies rapidly, destroying cells. Although the body's immune system attacks the viral organisms, some of them survive. The virus travels up nerve routes and entrenches itself in nerve cells. After that, the virus may remain inactive for weeks, months, or even years. When the virus isn't acting up, the body's defense system ignores it. However, if restimulated, the virus can become active again: it will retravel the nerve routes, reinfect cells, multiply again, and cause new sores to form. This cycle can repeat itself.

Treatment is aimed at relieving the symptoms of an attack, decreasing its length, avoiding complications, speeding the healing, and decreasing the frequency of recurrences.

Many different forms of treatment have been tried with little or no success. However, doctors have obtained promising results with the use of the amino acid lysine, taken orally in tablet form. Scientists are working to produce a vaccine.

- Zovirax

At present, the only medically accepted and effective treatment for genital herpes is the use of a prescription drug called acylovar, which is dispensed under the trade name Zovirax. It comes in both ointment and capsule form.

The only treatment
Zovirax doesn't eliminate the virus from the body and doesn't prevent transmission of the disease.

The ointment is effective for first-time attacks and relieves burning and itching. To prevent spreading the virus, wear rubber or plastic gloves when you apply this ointment. It should be applied to the affected area in the frequency recommended by your doctor; after

A vaccine
One such vaccine, called Lupidon, is used in Europe and reportedly prevents recurrences 90 to 95 percent of the time. This drug has not yet been approved for use in this country.

application, wash your gloves and hands thoroughly.

Zovirax capsules, which are used in short-term (5-day) or longer term (up to 6 months) therapy, can shorten the length of an attack, speed healing time of sores, prevent formation of new sores, and reduce the frequency of recurrence in 95 percent of herpes patients.

Because Zovirax capsules aren't given for longer than 6 months, a recurrence is likely when medication is stopped. Although the drug may cause side effects such as diarrhea, nausea, dizziness, and headache, such side effects aren't usually severe enough to force an end to the treatment.

- Aspirin

Aspirin or an aspirin substitute will help relieve the pain of herpes. Your doctor may also prescribe antihistamines, pain killers, or local anesthetics.

Prevention of herpes

Because herpes is highly contagious, people with an active outbreak of the disease should avoid sexual contact so as not to spread the virus.

The genital area should be kept thoroughly clean with soap and water and should be dried thoroughly after washing.

The body's own defenses should be maintained and bolstered with proper nutrition and adequate rest.

Warts

Warts are very common skin growths—millions of Americans have them—caused by a specific virus. Although they're unattractive, warts aren't symptoms of something worse and don't become cancerous. They can suddenly appear—and then just as suddenly disappear without treatment.

Warts are growths caused by a virus, and it's often emotional stress that activates the virus.

Plantar warts
Plantar warts are caused by the common wart virus. Since they usually appear on the points of pressure on the sole of your foot, they'll make walking painful or impossible, and you'll need immediate treatment for them.

Symptoms of warts

These unpopular growths come in several varieties.

- Common warts

Common warts can develop singly or in groups and may appear on any part of the body; they usually occur on the hands. Common warts are raised, have rough surfaces, are gray in color, and vary in size from as tiny as a matchhead to approximately an inch in diameter.

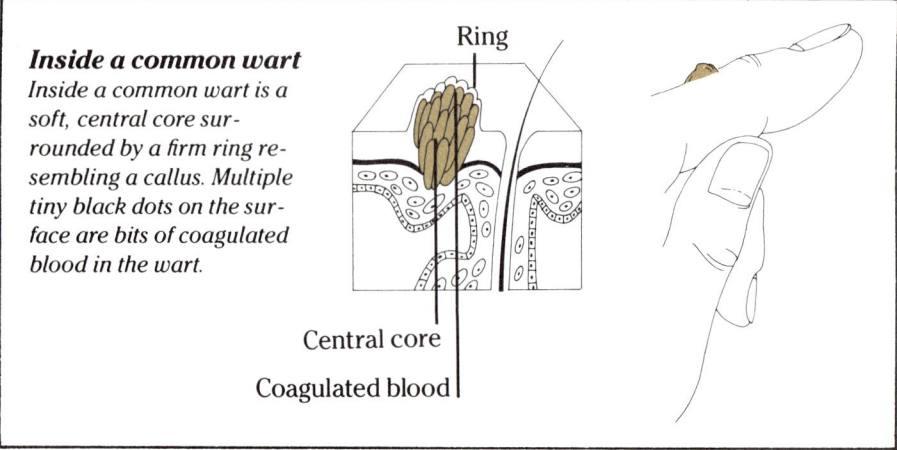

Inside a common wart
Inside a common wart is a soft, central core surrounded by a firm ring resembling a callus. Multiple tiny black dots on the surface are bits of coagulated blood in the wart.

Ring
Central core
Coagulated blood

Wart removers
The Food and Drug Administration studied wart removers for safety and effectiveness and had this to say: "Wart-remover drug products should not be used on moles, birthmarks, or unusual warts with hair growing from them because precancerous and cancerous growth may be mistaken for warts. Use of these products will aggravate these conditions. If treatment has not succeeded after 12 weeks, discontinue the over-the-counter medication and see a doctor."

- Flat warts

Flat warts are smooth and the color of skin. They're tiny, slightly raised growths and develop in a "spatter" pattern on the face, neck, chest, forearms, backs of the hands, and shins.

- Digitate warts

Digitate warts resemble fingerlike projections growing from a pea-shaped base. They develop in the scalp or near the hairline.

- Filiform warts

Filiform warts are long and narrow and occur on the neck and jaws.

- Genital warts

Genital warts develop in the moist areas around the sex organs and anus. These warts can be numerous and painful.

- Plantar warts

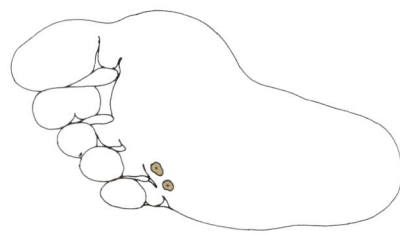

Plantar warts are large and occur on the soles of the feet. Because their surface is coarse and rough, they resemble corns and calluses. They're painful and resistant to treatment and are sometimes removed surgically if they make walking difficult.

Promising new treatment for genital warts

Interferon, a germ-fighting hormone, is being tested as a treatment for genital warts. Several treatments, including freezing, burning, and the use of caustic chemicals, are used now to remove genital warts, but more than half the time the warts come back. Interferon holds the promise of clearing up the warts permanently. Interferon is being tested as an injection into the wart itself.

Treatment for common warts

Common warts don't require treatment. Left to themselves, most warts will disappear spontaneously in a couple of years. You may want to get rid of them more quickly, particularly if they're causing pain.

If you're in a hurry:

1. Try a nonprescription wart medication, such as Duofilm or salicylic acid plaster.

2. If the wart is painful, see your doctor. He or she may use electrosurgery, freezing, chemicals, or surgery to remove the wart.

3. Hypnotism has proved helpful in getting rid of warts. The theory is that it may stimulate the body's immune system to reject the wart. Hypnotism is painless and leaves no scars.

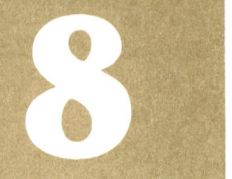

Common skin problems

Many skin problems aren't the result of accidents, disease, or infection. Although they may be distressing or displeasing, these common skin problems are normal and are experienced by most people.

Impetigo
This highly contagious skin infection is caused by two strains of bacteria—streptococcus and staphylococcus. Babies and children are most prone to impetigo because they haven't yet developed immunities to harmful bacteria. However, adults can also develop impetigo, usually by touching an infected child.

• Skin that has been damaged by an injury (such as a cut, abrasion, insect bite, scabies, or lice) or by a skin disorder (such as a cold sore, acne, or chicken pox) is unable to perform its job of keeping out harmful bacteria.

• Because they lower your resistance to infection, anemia and poor nutrition can make you susceptible to impetigo.

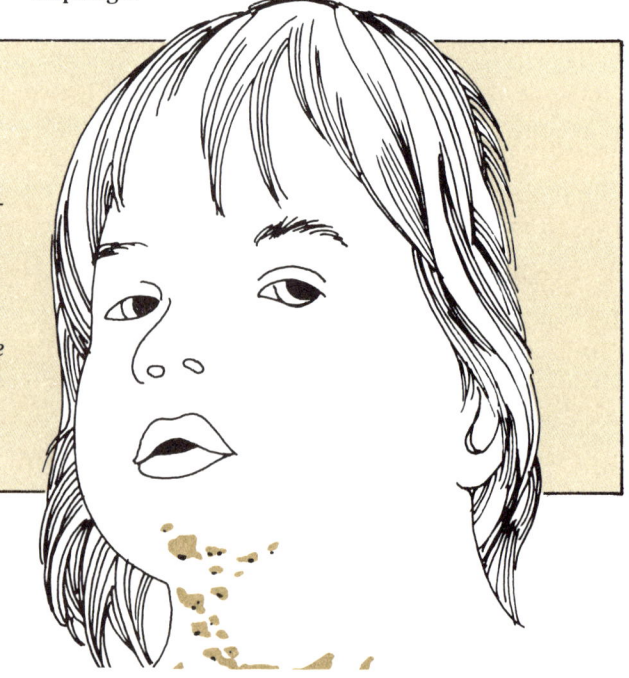

Impetigo
Don't pick, squeeze, or scratch skin infected with impetigo. The disease is highly contagious and easily spreads to other areas of the victim's body or to another person. Because impetigo is so contagious, an infected child should be kept away from other children (if possible) until his or her sores heal.

Skin safety for infants
The Food and Drug Administration has approved the following skin protectants for use on infants' skin without medical supervision:
- *allantoin*
- *aluminum hydroxide gel*
- *calamine*
- *cocoa butter*
- *cornstarch*
- *dimethicone*
- *glycerin*
- *petrolatum preparations (petrolatum, white petrolatum)*
- *sodium bicarbonate*
- *zinc carbonate*
- *zinc oxide*

All may be used on infants from birth except aluminum hydroxide gel and glycerin. You should wait until a child is six months old before using these products.

Phenol should never be used for diaper rash.

- Impetigo is highly contagious and easily transmitted. It can be spread by contact with discharged matter from the sores—either by direct contact or by means of towels, clothing, or similar objects that come in contact with the sores and are then handled by other people. Picking, squeezing, or scratching infected skin with fingernails can spread the disease to other people and can also spread the disease to other skin areas on an already infected person.

Symptoms of impetigo

The face, particularly around the mouth and nose, the arms and legs, the scalp, and hands are the most common locations, but any part of the body may become infected.

- Blisters appear and increase in size and number. They may be filled with a watery fluid or with thick yellow pus.

- As the blisters break, thick yellow-brown crusts develop and adhere to the affected skin. These may itch.

- If not treated and eliminated, impetigo can spread, enlarging the infected area. It can also, of course, be spread to other people.

- Impetigo can result in a secondary infection (affecting internal organs), involving pain, fever, and other symptoms of illness.

Treatment for impetigo

To prevent the spread of impetigo, the infected person should cleanse the area around the sores frequently. The infected person should also wash his or her hands frequently and should avoid touching or scratching the sores. To cleanse:

1. Wash the area several times a day with warm water and soap.

2. Apply warm water or tepid saltwater compresses to soften the crusts on the blisters.

3. Gently wash the loosened crusts off the skin with soap and water.

4. Apply antiseptic or antibacterial ointments.

5. Continue these procedures for 1 week after the crusts have fallen off.

Prevention of impetigo

- Avoid direct contact with anyone with signs of impetigo.

A common skin problem for babies

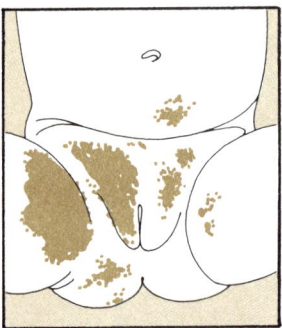

Diaper rash can make babies uncomfortable and unhappy.

Call your pediatrician
If diaper rash or prickly heat doesn't clear up in a couple of days, call your pediatrician. The rash may be the symptom of a medical problem such as a milk allergy.

- Practice good skin hygiene, being particularly careful to keep your hands and fingernails thoroughly clean.

- Don't use another person's towel or washcloth and don't share clothing.

- If someone in your household is infected, launder his or her clothing, linens, towels, and washcloths apart from the family wash.

Diaper rash and prickly heat

These common skin disorders are usually associated with babies, and although neither is dangerous, both can result in serious bacterial and fungal infections if untreated. Fortunately, both are easily preventable.

Causes of diaper rash

Diaper rash produces reddening and soreness of a baby's skin in the areas usually covered by a diaper. This skin irritation develops on a baby's buttocks, in the anal area, around the genitals, on the upper thighs, and on the lower abdomen. Usually caused by wet diapers, it tends to recur.

- Lack of ventilation in the susceptible body areas keeps skin moist and inhibits the natural breathing process of the skin; combined with the moisture of wet diapers, this can lead to diaper rash.

- Heat and humidity keep skin overly moist, clog sweat pores, and result in inflammation. Interference with the skin's normal functions encourages the growth of bacteria and fungi.

- Anything that further irritates the baby's delicate skin—detergents, fabric softeners, bleaches, soaps, baby oils, ointments—can worsen diaper rash. The noxious intestinal enzymes produced when the baby has diarrhea will also worsen the rash.

Symptoms of diaper rash

- Skin becomes reddened and chafed.

- Tiny pimples and blisters appear.

- When these blisters break, the area becomes moist and smells of ammonia; sometimes open sores appear.

Irritants to baby's skin
Detergents, fabric softeners (especially perfumed ones), and bleaches used in laundering diapers can all cause allergic reactions in addition to diaper rash.

Treatment and prevention of diaper rash

1. Apply compresses soaked in Burow's solution or Domeboro powder solution every 3 hours to soothe the inflammation and irritation.
2. Apply a medicated nonprescription ointment.
3. Change diapers as soon as they become wet or soiled.
4. Don't use plastic or rubber diaper coverings during the night.
5. After each diaper change, thoroughly cleanse the area prone to rash, including the small skin folds.
6. Use mild soap—but no soap at all when the area is inflamed.
7. After washing, thoroughly dry the area.
8. Sprinkle on a specially medicated powder or baby powder; cornstarch works well.
9. Keep the baby's clothing loose enough to allow air circulation in the area.

Causes of prickly heat

Prickly heat, also called heat rash, is caused by heat—hot climate, inner body fever, high humidity, overdressing in cool weather—that causes excessive, prolonged sweating. This can interfere with the flow from the skin's more than 2 million sweat glands. The overworked ducts become blocked, preventing the proper evaporation of sweat. Babies and young children are most commonly affected.

Wearing too-tight clothing compounds the problem by increasing perspiration and making normal sweat evaporation difficult.

Symptoms of prickly heat

- Rash that forms tiny red pimples
- Itching and burning
- Sometimes, the sweat trapped in the closed pores may cause a bacterial or fungal infection resulting in large pus-filled sores.

Treatment for prickly heat

1. Avoid becoming overheated; try to keep your skin cool and dry.
2. Sprinkle your skin with a cornstarch-based powder.

Eczema

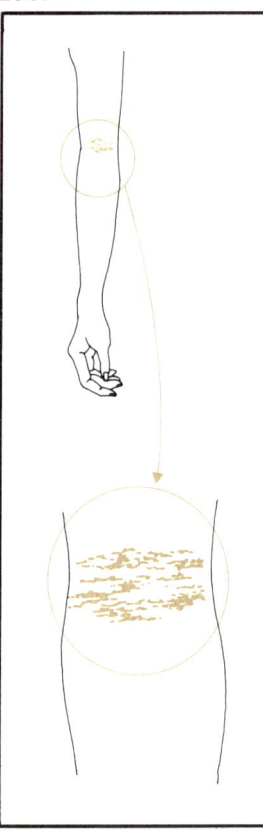

Eczema is a common skin problem that produces crusty, thick scales. Children and adults can get eczema, but the later in life it occurs, the more severe the symptoms.

The cause of eczema is unknown, but it's thought to be allergy related.

3. Avoid greasy creams or ointments. These cause additional pore-clogging.

4. Take frequent cool or tepid showers, baths, or sponge baths.

5. Wear minimal, loose, and lightweight clothing. Don't overdress in cold weather.

6. Take advantage of air-conditioning or fans.

7. If your symptoms persist or worsen, consult your doctor. Secondary infections resulting from prickly heat can be dangerous.

Eczema

Eczema, also called dermatitis, is a common, noncontagious skin eruption that almost always appears first in infancy.

Causes of eczema

- The inflammation and rash are believed to be due to an inherited allergic sensitivity to one or more substances. This sensitivity is present from birth and may remain throughout your life.

- Exposure to the offending substance will cause an outbreak of eczema.

- In addition to foods (particularly wheat, milk, and eggs), clothing made from animal components (such as fur, wool, feathers, silk), dust, perfumes, and detergents are common offenders.

- Emotional stress is probably a contributing factor, as it is in any allergic-type disorder.

- Excessive perspiration that doesn't evaporate is another cause.

- Extremes of temperature and humidity aggravate eczema.

Symptoms of eczema

- A persistent, itching, inflammatory eruption of the skin is present. It may be an acute outbreak or it may be chronic.

- Eczema tends to recur unless the responsible substance is eliminated.

- Eczema may become linked to asthma or hay fever.

- The symptoms on the skin are rash, redness, scaling or crusting blisters, swelling, and breaks in the skin.

- Occasionally, there's an oozing of watery fluid.

Eczema can occur at different ages. Because the sensitivity is inherited, a baby is susceptible to eczema from birth. Within the first couple of months to the age of 2, the red eruption may appear (on the face, cheeks, neck, inner surfaces of elbows and knees) accompanied by intense itching.

From 2 to 4, a child's eczema may recur, but if the child has not yet had it, it may appear for the first time. The most frequent locations of the eruption are the inner surfaces of the elbows and knees. The skin becomes thickened, and the rash is gray, rather than red. Severe itching causes restlessness and irritability.

Eczema that disappeared in childhood may recur in late adolescence and persist for several years or even a lifetime. Although the most frequent locations are the inner surfaces of the elbows and knees, the face, shoulders, and back may also be affected. Itching is intense, particularly at night. The skin becomes thickened, discolored, and scaly.

Treatment for eczema

1. Try to identify and eliminate the offending substance; this may be a certain food, pet, dust, chemical, kind of clothing, carpet, or even a favorite teddy bear.

2. Keep emotional stress at as low a level as possible.

3. Avoid excessive sweating and extremes of temperature.

4. Take an antihistamine to relieve itching.

5. Apply compresses moistened with Domeboro or Blueboro powder solution during the oozing stage of eczema. This will reduce inflammation and relieve itching.

6. Apply medicated nonprescription creams and lotions.

7. For chronic eczema with dry, scaly skin, apply a nonprescription medicated lubricating cream or ointment.

8. If you have eczema, avoid soap; instead, cleanse with nonprescription eczema cleansers and eczema shampoos.

9. Avoid contact with people who have cold sores or have had recent smallpox vaccinations; the virus responsible for these conditions can cause dangerous skin infections.

10. For a severe eczema eruption, consult your doctor. He or she may prescribe an oral or injected steroid-type drug, a tar-based ointment, cream, or lotion, or ultraviolet B light therapy.

Athlete's foot
Athlete's foot is a fungal infection. It may be contracted in public shower rooms or result from your feet being cooped up in moist places for too long.

Athlete's foot
Athlete's foot is a fungal infection that usually affects the feet; it may affect any other part of the body, such as the scalp, under the nails, or the palms of the hands.

Causes of athlete's foot
Fungi cause athlete's foot. These are tiny organisms that under a microscope look much like plants and can grow on our skin, hair, and nails.

Although fungi are always present on your feet, you won't develop athlete's foot unless the fungi find the necessary conditions for growth. These conditions include excessive moisture, lack of cleanliness, insufficient air circulation, or an abrasion to the skin.

Because it increases sweating, emotional tension may spur the growth of fungi.

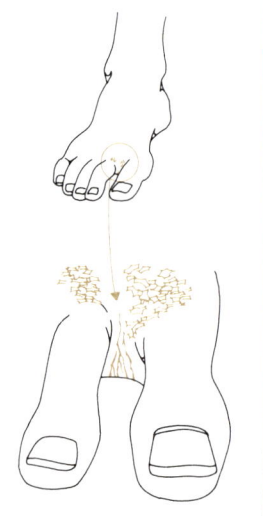

Who gets athlete's foot?
Perhaps because they sweat more, wear heavier, more confining shoes and socks (which permit less ventilation), or even because of hormonal differences or different hygiene habits, men are more prone to athlete's foot than are women. However, being athletic is unrelated to developing this infection—except that athletic activity creates additional sweating.

Symptoms of athlete's foot
• Scaling, blisters, and peeling occur between the toes (particularly the smaller toes). The infection may also be present on the soles of the feet.

• There is often severe itching.

• If the disease progresses, pain and inflammation may also be present.

• The fungus will spread; as it does so, the open sores at the site of the original infection will begin to heal. A red ring marks the spread of the fungus and the infection.

- Round patches of scaly, red skin develop. These vary in size from that of a pinhead to a half-dollar.

Treatment for athlete's foot

1. While the sores or blisters are open and oozing, soak your feet every 4 hours in either Domeboro or Blueboro powder solution.

2. When the sores begin to dry out, apply antifungal creams or sprays.

3. Use an antifungal powder.

4. Keep infected toes separated with strips of soft cotton fabric; never use cotton balls because they can be irritating due to their wood-fiber content.

5. Because athlete's foot attacks soft, weak skin, you can use a skin toughener such as Onox to help prevent recurrences.

6. Wear only cotton socks, preferably white, and boil them after every use.

7. If your infection hasn't cleared up in 2 to 3 weeks, consult your doctor. You may require an antibiotic drug to fight a secondary bacterial infection that may have developed. Or you may have mistaken psoriasis or an allergic dermatitis for athlete's foot.

8. For a persistent or spreading athlete's foot infection that doesn't subside by means of the suggested home treatments, your doctor will probably prescribe an oral antifungal medication.

Prevention of athlete's foot

- Go barefoot whenever possible and safe, particularly during the warm months of the summer. Keep your feet cool and dry.

- Wash your feet daily and dry them thoroughly, especially between the toes.

- Wear shoes that "breathe"—leather rather than vinyl. Sandals and sneakers are preferable to closed shoes.

Canker sores

Canker sores are small, ulcerated sores that usually appear on the inside of the mouth, on the gums, palate, or sides of the tongue. They're often confused with cold sores, but unlike cold sores, canker sores aren't caused by a virus. Nor are they contagious, hereditary, or cancer-related. But they're very painful and resistant to treatment.

Although canker sores heal by themselves within a week or two, they tend to recur, sometimes frequently, in persons prone to them—and an estimated 20 to 50 percent of the population is prone to them.

Possible causes of canker sores

The exact cause of canker sores isn't known, but certain factors seem to trigger an outbreak:

• Damaged or irritated skin inside the mouth; biting the inside of the cheek or the irritation caused by dental operations

• A sensitivity to certain foods such as citrus fruits, chocolate, sodas, spices, and milk

• Nutritional deficiencies, particularly in iron, folic acid, and Vitamin B_{12}

• Physical or emotional stress

• Allergies

• Bacteria and viruses that aren't controlled by proper mouth hygiene

---

Cold sores and canker sores—what's the difference?

Don't confuse cold sores with canker sores. Canker sores appear inside the mouth as white spots with a red ring around them. The Food and Drug Administration reviewed over-the-counter products for the treatment of canker sores and found that none work.

Always contact your doctor if you suspect a canker sore.

Cold sores are around the mouth or on the lips and are red, painful, and unattractive. Like canker sores, they're generally unresponsive to medicine. Neither can be cured, but both will go away at their own rate.

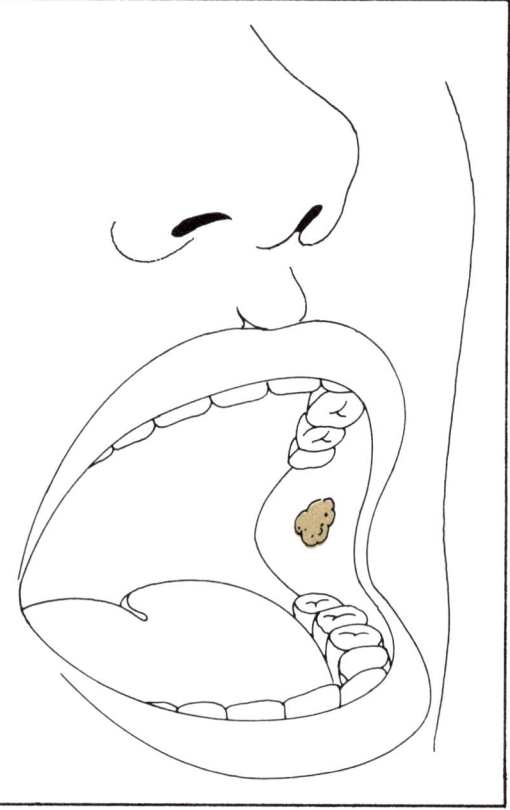

Temporary relief
Nonprescription canker sore medications won't heal canker sores and will only relieve the pain for a few minutes by numbing the area. For longer relief, you'll have to reapply the medicine every 20 minutes or so.

Symptoms of canker sores
- Small blisters or eruptions in the mouth.
- These are followed by larger sores—oval and yellowish with a red rim—that become swollen and painful.

Treatment for canker sores
1. Rinsing the mouth with a mild solution of one teaspoonful of table salt to a pint of warm water may help soothe the irritation.
2. Apply a nonprescription canker sore medication such as Ambesol First Aid for Canker Sores or Campho-Phenique.
3. Apply a moistened tea bag or an ice cube to the sore.
4. For persistent or recurrent canker sores, consult your doctor. He or she may prescribe an antibiotic such as tetracycline to be used as a mouth rinse (it's held in the mouth for 2 or 3 minutes before being swallowed). Your doctor may also prescribe vitamin and iron supplements.

Prevention of canker sores
1. Try to detect specific foods that may be triggering an outbreak and avoid them.
2. Practice good mouth and dental hygiene.
3. If you wear dentures, be sure they fit properly.
4. Make a habit of eating yogurt; it seems to suppress the development of canker sores.

Psoriasis
Psoriasis is a mystery disease. It's not life-threatening or life-shortening, and it's not contagious. It isn't related to an allergy, an infection, or poor nutrition. It develops with equal frequency in both sexes and can occur at any age, but it appears most frequently between the ages of 15 and 35.

Psoriasis is a chronic skin disease that creates enough misery among its sufferers—more than 8 million in the United States—to cause them to spend $1 billion a year in search of relief.

We know a number of things about what psoriasis isn't, but we know very little about its causes and treatment. Indeed, the most certain fact about psoriasis is that it's usually incurable.

Psoriasis

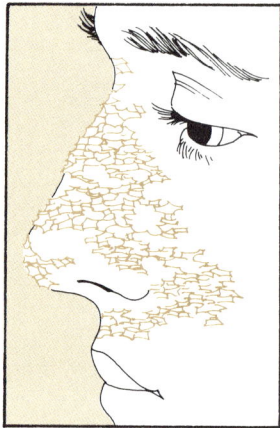

Psoriasis is a common skin disorder. It's characterized by red patches covered by thick, dry, silvery scales. These scales are the result of skin cells dividing too rapidly.

Possible causes of psoriasis

• Hereditary factors are believed to be related to psoriasis, but the evidence isn't clearly established. We do know that psoriasis tends to run in some families.

• Although the precise cause remains a mystery, suspected triggers include skin damage (cut, burn, or scrape); some forms of infection (such as severe upper respiratory infection or strep throat in children); certain chemical disturbances within the body; physical stress; pregnancy; hormonal imbalances; certain foods; and medications used to treat other diseases.

• Emotional stress appears to be a precipitating factor.

• Seasonal changes may affect the severity of psoriasis. The disease responds well to sunlight; but a sunburn can cause it.

Although the cause or causes of psoriasis are still uncertain, we do know the process of the disease. Psoriasis results from an abnormality in the growth and reproduction of skin cells. The process by which the skin normally develops an outer layer and then discards the worn-out cells becomes disordered. Instead of the cells on the skin's outer layer shedding about every 27 days after they're formed, the rate of cell formation in psoriasis accelerates 10 times; the skin begins to shed cells every 4 or 5 days. This abnormal multiplication causes a buildup of cells in a thickened accumulation on the skin surface.

Symptoms of psoriasis

• Patches of silvery gray scales covering red sores appear.

• There are clearly defined red borders between the patches and normal skin.

• The patches of scales may be very tiny or large enough to cover large areas of the body.

• The patches usually appear on the elbows, knees, trunk, and scalp but can occur on any skin area (the palms of the hands and soles of the feet are other common locations).

• The appearance of the patches may vary slightly, according to the site. Elbows, knees, chest, abdomen, and back develop thick, red scaling patches; the scalp develops red patches with sharp borders visible at the hairline—large amounts of silver scales, resembling dandruff, are shed from these patches. When psoriasis affects the nails, they may become pitted and lose their shine. The genital area may develop painful red sores that may preclude sexual relations.

• There may be itching.

• If the condition becomes acute, there may be painful reddening of the entire skin, accompanied by cracking and shedding of the skin around the joints along with chills. This form of psoriasis often requires hospitalization and treatment.

• Because of the embarrassment accompanying this unsightly skin disease, severe emotional trauma may result.

• Although psoriasis is chronic, its pattern is to improve, even disappear, for a time and then to reappear intermittently, perhaps in an even worse form. Between attacks, the skin regains a normal appearance, with no scaling.

Treatment for psoriasis

1. Apply baby oil or petroleum jelly to the scales to soften them.

2. Bathe in special nonprescription preparations with a tar base (but only if you're not allergic to tar). This relieves itching and reduces scaling.

3. Use medicated nonprescription psoriasis soaps, ointments, and shampoos (be alert for allergic reactions to these products).

4. Apply a steroid-type cream several times a day— after bathing and at night—to relieve itching.

5. Covering your skin with plastic wrap, plastic gloves, or a vinyl exercise suit, after bathing or after applying a cream or ointment, often produces excellent results in eliminating sores and scaling.

6. Take a nonprescription antihistamine every 4 hours if needed to relieve itching.

7. Many psoriasis sufferers experience improvement if they expose the affected area to sunlight or the light of an ultraviolet lamp.

8. Carefully observe the effect of foods you eat to determine which may aggravate your psoriasis— eliminate these foods. Meat, seafood, alcoholic drinks, and some medications taken for other ailments have been cited as offenders.

9. If these measures don't provide adequate relief,

An arthritis-psoriasis link?
There's indication that a form of arthritis, resulting in joint disease and pain, may be associated with a flare-up of psoriasis.

or if your psoriasis is severe, consult your doctor. Cortisone-steroid drugs in oral or injected form can prove effective in reducing symptoms. Also helpful are prescribed ointments composed of tar-sulphur-allantoin-salicylic acid ingredients (these are particularly good if they're applied to the affected area and then covered with plastic wrap during the night). PUVA treatment, in which an oral dose of the drug methoxalen is followed by ultraviolet light exposure, has also produced very encouraging results because it slows down the abnormal multiplication process and prevents additional scale formation.

Lice

Lice are tiny parasitic insects. When viewed through a microscope, body lice resemble minute lobsters, and head and pubic lice resemble minute crabs. Once you've seen them, it becomes clear why this form of infestation is called crabs.

Lice attach themselves to people. Head lice attach themselves to the scalp; pubic lice to the pubic hairs and skin in the pubic area; body lice to clothing (they move to the skin only to feed). Lice nourish themselves on human blood. They bite into the skin and suck out blood; at the same time, they inject a toxic substance that causes itching and possibly an allergic reaction, fever, headache, or general "sick" feeling. Worst of all, lice (particularly body lice) are carriers of typhus, a serious infectious disease that affects the nervous system and is accompanied by a rash and high fever.

Causes of lice infestations

- Lice are transmitted by direct contact with infested persons, their clothing, bed linens, towels, combs, and brushes. You can come in contact with lice anywhere an infected person has undressed or slept. Pubic lice are commonly transmitted during sexual relations.

- Crowded and dirty living conditions and poor personal hygiene contribute to the spread of the infestation.

- Anyone, no matter how clean and fastidious, can become infested with lice simply by brushing against a carrier.

Itching
Itching is worse at night because lice are more active in a warm environment such as that presented by a warm body in a warm bed.

Symptoms of lice infestations

Head lice can be observed as small ovals of grayish-white or silvery nits (eggs) attached to hair shafts very close to the scalp. They're firmly attached by means of a sticky substance secreted by the female lice.

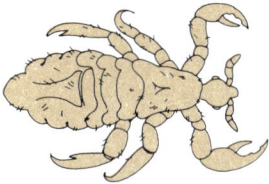

Head lice

They produce small red bites on the scalp, back of the head and neck, and behind the ears. Intense itching is present. Scratching the itch results in marks on the skin.

There may also be a rash on the chest and abdomen caused by a reaction to the louse toxin injected into the scalp when a louse bites.

In severe cases, the lymph glands in the neck swell, and the hair may be matted, foul-smelling, and dull in color. There may be sores and, later, scarring.

Pubic lice can be observed as nits and rust-colored adults attached to hair in the pubic area. Occasionally, pubic lice attach themselves to the eyelashes, eyebrows, or armpit hairs.

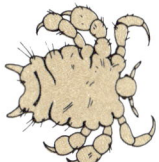

Pubic lice

Lice bites can be seen in the region of the genitals, abdomen, and lower thighs.

There is intense itching, particularly at night. Marks on the skin are often present from scratching the itch. Grayish-blue marks may appear on the trunk and thighs. In severe cases, fever and swollen lymph glands may occur.

Body lice can be detected by the bites on the areas of the body that come in contact with infested clothing. These appear most frequently on the shoulders, in the armpits, and around the waist. A red rash may appear on the shoulders, back, abdomen, and buttocks.

Itching and resultant scratch marks are other symptoms.

If neglected, the infestation may produce dry, discolored scaly skin with thick crusts and bacterial infection. Scarring may result.

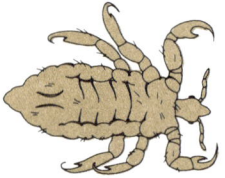

Body lice

In severe cases, there may be fever, headache, and a "sick" feeling.

Treatment for lice infestations

1. Head lice can be eliminated by washing the hair and scalp with a prescription shampoo called Kwell.
2. Nonprescription anti-lice shampoos, such as Rid, are also effective.
3. Kwell cream or lotion (by prescription) can be applied and left on the skin for 8 to 12 hours.
4. After shampooing or applying a cream or lotion, the dead nits and lice can be loosened from the hair shafts by applying a solution of half vinegar and half water.
5. Comb the hair, using a fine-tooth comb dipped in vinegar to remove the rest of the dead lice.
6. To get rid of body lice and pubic lice, use medicated soaps and water. For severe cases, apply Kwell lotion or cream. Leave it on for 8 to 12 hours.
7. Launder (in very hot water) or dry clean any articles of clothing, sheets, pillow cases, blankets, mattress covers, or towels that may be infested. Pay attention to seams, for lice tend to locate in them.
8. Avoid sharing any possibly infested hats, combs, hair brushes, clothing, headbands, pillow cases, or scarves.
9. Wear and use only freshly laundered or dry cleaned clothing and linens.

Scabies

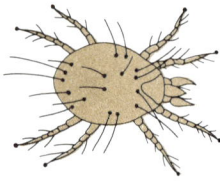

Scabie
This illustration of a scabie is greatly enlarged. A scabie can be identified only when it's seen under a microscope.

Many skin disorders cause itching, but scabies takes the prize for producing a maddening itch (which is worse at night) and an almost uncontrollable urge to scratch.

Scabies is common and can be picked up by anyone, no matter how fastidious the person might be. Each year 2 million Americans are affected by this skin disorder.

Scabies is caused by a mite, a tiny, insectlike creature related to ticks. The mite that causes scabies is known as the itch mite. These insects are so tiny they're barely visible without the use of a magnifying glass.

The itch mites that cause scabies live under the skin of the humans they infest. The female itch mite burrows into and under the upper layers of skin, creating tunnels. She deposits her eggs in these tunnels. The eggs hatch in 3 to 5 days, and the young itch mites also tunnel under the skin. They emerge from the skin to mate, and then burrow again. This process continues.

The burrowing, tunneling, and excretion of the itch mites produce the agonizing itch of scabies.

Causes of scabies

- Overcrowded and unsanitary living conditions and inadequate personal hygiene contribute to the spread of scabies, but anyone can get it—scabies is transmitted by contact with an infected person. The itch mites on the skin surface of an infected person can spread easily to the skin of another person.

- Children are apt to develop scabies from hand-to-hand contact, sharing of clothing, and touching of infested pets (particularly puppies). Children then spread the infestation to the rest of the family or to other children.

Symptoms of scabies

- Intense, excruciating itching is the primary characteristic of scabies. This itching is worse at night.

- Because of this nighttime itching, sleeplessness, irritability, and nervousness may accompany scabies.

- Although any part of the body below chin level may be affected, itch mites prefer to burrow into these areas: between the fingers, backs of the hands, armpits, inner surfaces of the wrists, the back of the elbows, the shoulder blades, around the navel, the waist, buttocks, nipples, genitals, and ankles.

- Diagnosis is often difficult because the infestation

may be confused with contact dermatitis or eczema because of the rash and itching.

- What may appear to be a rash are actually the burrows, gray-white, raised and threadlike, in a zigzag pattern resembling scratches. At the end of a burrow there may be a tiny blister and small sore that appears as a reddened or black dotlike pimple.
- Scratching the itch may open the skin and cause a secondary bacterial infection.

Treatment for scabies

1. To be certain of the diagnosis of scabies, you should consult your doctor. A sample of the skin, scraped off and examined by microscope, may be necessary to confirm the presence of eggs, itch mites, and their excretions.

2. A traditional and effective treatment for scabies in infants is sulphur ointment. However, this is greasy, messy, has a very unpleasant odor, and stains clothing.

3. Kwell or Eurax cream or lotion, commercial products prepared with the chemical lindane, are used by doctors in the treatment of scabies. Neither has the unpleasant or uncomfortable qualities of the old-time sulphur remedy. Both, however, must be prescribed by a doctor. They should be used exactly as instructed or other skin ailments may result.

- Before using one of these preparations, you should take a lengthy soap and warm water bath.
- After the bath, let your body cool down and air dry.
- Apply a thin layer of the Kwell or Eurax cream or lotion to your entire body from the neck down and rub it into the skin.
- Repeat the treatment after 12 to 24 hours.

4. Because scabies is so easily transmitted, all family members and sexual partners should undergo treatment. They may have scabies even though they're not suffering symptoms: symptoms may take several weeks to appear.

5. If you have any secondary bacterial infection, your doctor will prescribe an antibiotic.

Large pores

A pore is an opening on the skin's surface marking a sweat gland, oil gland, or hair follicle. Each of us has millions of pores. The size of these pores varies from person to person and is a hereditary characteristic: some people have small pores; some have large ones.

In addition, pore sizes differ from one part of the body to another. A great number of oil glands are located on your face, in such areas as the nose, cheeks, chin, and lips. These pores may become extended because of the oil produced in the oil glands. Thus, large facial pores aren't an abnormality—they're just an individual physical trait.

Causes of large pores
Various conditions can exaggerate your pores' appearance:

• Adolescent acne can "stretch" the oil ducts, enlarging pores.

• Pores that are full of oil, as happens in excessively oily skin, appear larger.

• Squeezing pimples or blackheads has a scarring effect that can permanently distend pores.

Treatment for large pores
No product can change the size of your pores. However, you can prevent oil from accumulating in your pores:

• Wash thoroughly
Make it a practice to thoroughly cleanse your skin with soap and warm water. This will inhibit oil buildup in your pores.

• Use oil-free or water-based cosmetics
Oil-free or water-based cosmetics won't contribute additional oil to your skin.

• Use only light moisturizers
Use of a light, rather than heavy, moisturizer will also help prevent the accumulation of oil on your skin.

Wrinkles
Wrinkles are normal, inevitable accompaniments to aging. With each passing decade a person's skin becomes thinner and dryer. In youth, the process is slow and indiscernible, but by the time we reach our mid-thirties, our skin has become less elastic, less flexible, and thinner. Lines begin to form.

Causes of wrinkles
Several factors contribute to the formation of wrinkles. Some of these are beyond your control—they're natural results of aging; others are within your control.

Dispelling a myth
Dry skin doesn't cause wrinkles, and it usually corrects itself when the weather turns warm and humidity increases.

Wrinkles

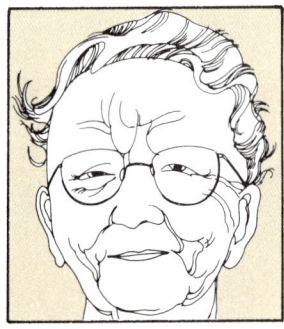

Wrinkles are natural, but you may be surprised by the number of factors that cause them. Eleven are listed here.

The factors contributing to wrinkles that are beyond your control include:

- Loss of lubrication

As the years pass, our oil and sweat glands, which have worked to moisturize our skin and keep it smooth and supple, decrease in size and number. Losing this constant supply of lubrication, skin starts to dry out and wrinkle.

- Sagging skin

The collagen and elastic fibers that support skin weaken with time. As a result, skin begins to sag.

- Loss of elasticity

As hormone production decreases, skin is deprived of its benefits. Beneath the skin's surface, fat shrinks and fibrous tissue connecting the skin to muscles becomes weak and flabby, allowing the skin to "cave in" and wrinkle.

- Heredity

Ethnic groups that are fair in complexion, such as the Irish, English, and Scandinavians, are prone to earlier wrinkling than are dark-skinned ethnic groups.

Those factors about which you can do something include:

- Exposure to the sun

Exposure to the sun (and extreme cold, heat, or wind) accelerates the aging of your skin. Avoiding the damage done to skin by the sun is of the utmost importance and is completely within your control. If you work outdoors, always wear a sunscreen.

- Crash diets

Crash diets or alternating weight gain and loss cause the skin to lose its underlying foundation and form. With less fat and muscle underneath, the skin hangs in loose, baggy folds—and becomes wrinkled. Avoid drastic changes in your weight.

- Facial exercises

Facial exercises, often recommended to prevent wrinkles, can weaken the skin's elastic fibers and actually cause wrinkles.

- Facial contortions

Excessive frowning, rough massages, or any exaggerated and constant grimacing (such as that of smokers squinting to avoid getting smoke in their eyes) can contribute to wrinkles.

- Smoking
Heavy smokers suffer decreased blood supply, which compounds the wrinkling problem. If you smoke, try to quit—avoiding wrinkles is only one of the many reasons to do so.

- Excessive washing
Too frequent washing, especially with hot water and soap, deprives skin of its natural oils and may also weaken its elastic fibers. Use gentle soaps and cleansers and warm, not hot, water for washing your skin.

- Improper diet
Improper diet over a long period doesn't supply adequate nutrition to maintain healthy skin. Make proper nutrition, including adequate vitamin, mineral, and fluid intake, part of your life.

Treatment for wrinkles

- Moisturize your skin
Moisturize and lubricate your skin with substitutes for your body's natural oils. Use any of a great variety of oils and creams with animal extracts, plant extracts, and chemical formulas. These are "poor cousins" compared to your body's natural oils, but they're better than nothing in helping alleviate dryness, roughness, and cracking—all of which can cause wrinkles.

- Facial masks
Facial masks can have a temporary firming effect.

- Remove wrinkles surgically
Surgery performed by a qualified plastic or cosmetic surgeon can—if successful—perform wonderful feats of reversing the inroads of time. However, the results of this type of surgery are sometimes disappointing. These procedures can be painful and expensive, and they don't last indefinitely. To maintain the new look, the surgery must be repeated at intervals of approximately 5 years.

Dry skin

If your skin feels or looks tight, rough, flaky, or itchy, you have what is commonly referred to as dry skin. This condition isn't necessarily associated with aging, and although it's more prevalent among older people, there are various other causes.

Considering a lift?
While a facelift or eyelift can't remove years from your age, it can make you look and feel younger. For some people, expense and discomfort are small considerations compared to the morale boost that such surgery—if successful—offers.

Moisture robbers
Cold air and lower humidity draw moisture from the cells in the outer layers of your skin.... In the absence of perspiration, your skin is unable to bring moisture from its inner layers to its surface.

Causes of dry skin
• Heredity
Some ethnic groups are more prone to dry skin than others. In general, fair-skinned people suffer more from dry skin than do dark-skinned people.
• Exposure to the elements
Exposure to the sun, wind, and cold can all contribute to dry skin.
• Washing
The use of soaps containing alkali and bathing or washing your face with hot water may dry your skin.
• Harsh laundry detergents
Even if you have normal skin, it may become dry if it's in frequent contact with clothing, sheets, pillow cases, and towels that have been laundered in harsh detergents and not properly rinsed.
• Clothing
Heavy woolen or rough clothing may also irritate skin.
• Dry air
Spending time in rooms warmed by furnaces, hot-air vents, "forced air," or other heating devices can dry skin. These extract moisture from the air, indoor plants, and your skin. Because of this, dry skin is particularly common during the winter.

Treatment for dry skin
• Use emollient creams, lotions, and oils to lubricate and moisturize your skin. These, and whatever natural oils are on your skin, help to prevent further loss of moisture. They keep your skin smoother, softer, and more elastic.

• After your shower, spray your skin (while it's still moist) with a lubricating body oil. As moisturizers do for your hands, this oil forms a protective moisture "seal" on your body, locking moisture in your skin's cells. If you take baths rather than showers, use warm, not hot, water to which bath oils have been added. This, too, will provide a protective coating of moisture for your skin.

• Use soaps and skin cleansers that are formulated to restore oil to your skin.

Moles
Moles are the most common skin tumors and are medically called nevi (one mole is a nevus). In nonmedical terminology, moles are often called birthmarks or beauty marks.

Changes in a mole

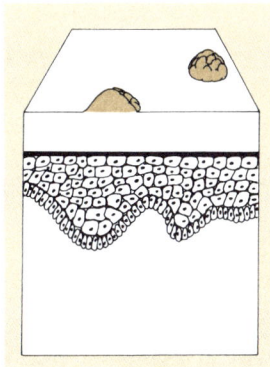

Watch for suspicious changes in your skin. Such changes may be early warning symptoms of cancer. Fortunately, spotting changes isn't difficult once you get to know your body and what's normal for it. Watch for these changes:
• *Asymmetry.* Most skin cancers are asymmetrical. If you drew a line down the center of a cancerous growth, the two halves wouldn't match.
• *Border.* The borders of skin cancers are often notched or uneven, while those of normal moles or freckles are usually even or smooth.
• *Color.* A skin cancer may contain mixed shades of several colors, unlike a normal mark, which is usually all one color.
• *Diameter.* A skin cancer is usually wider than a pencil eraser, making it larger than most normal freckles or moles.
  Skin cancers are easy to cure. Indeed, early detection and treatment of skin cancer virtually guarantee its cure.

The cause of moles is unknown, but they tend to run in families.

Symptoms of moles
• Most moles appear during adolescence; they often disappear with age.
• Moles vary greatly in appearance. They may be flat or raised; hairless or hairy. Their colors vary, too, from pale pink to dark brown.

Treatment for moles
No treatment is required for most moles. It sometimes becomes desirable to remove moles for cosmetic reasons or because their size or location is a source of irritation (a mole may make shaving difficult).

Moles may become darker or more numerous due to hormonal changes during adolescence, pregnancy, or menopause.

Consult your doctor if any mole increases in size, bleeds without injury, changes in color, changes in texture, or changes in feeling (becomes itchy or painful). Such changes may indicate the development of a malignant growth such as a melanoma.

Upon examining you, your doctor may do one or more of the following:
1. Perform a biopsy (microscopic examination of a small sample of the tissue) to determine whether or not the tissue is malignant.
2. Remove the mole surgically.
3. Use electrosurgery (which sears the blood vessels shut so that any cancer cells that may be present aren't freed into the bloodstream) combined with curette surgery (using a sharp ring-shaped instrument) to remove a tumor.

Keratoses
There are two types of these skin lesions. One is seborrheic keratoses, which is harmless. The other is actinic keratoses, which is an early form of skin cancer and is discussed in the next chapter.

Seborrheic keratoses
The cause of seborrheic keratoses is unknown, but they seem to develop with age.

Symptoms of seborrheic keratoses
• Seborrheic keratoses are tan, brown, or black

Keratoses

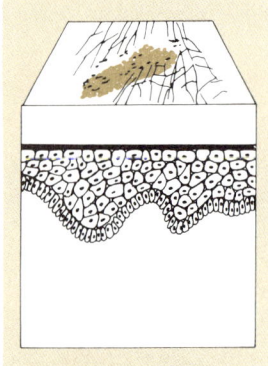

There are two types of these skin lesions. One is seborrheic keratoses, which is harmless. The other is actinic keratoses, which is an early form of skin cancer and is discussed in the next chapter.

growths; they're usually slightly raised and have a waxy, crusted surface.

- They appear to be "stuck on" or loosely attached to the skin.
- They occur most frequently on the back and chest and, occasionally, on the face.
- They may be very tiny or over an inch in diameter, and they vary in shape. They grow slowly.
- They usually appear after age 40.

Treatment for seborrheic keratoses

No treatment is necessary for seborrheic keratoses. If for cosmetic or medical reasons you want or need to remove them, your doctor will use one of these methods:

1. Curette surgery: the area is numbed with a local anesthetic and the growth is then scraped off with a curette (a sharp ring-shaped instrument).

2. Electrosurgery, which is also performed after a local anesthetic is applied: an electric current directed through a needle burns the growth, which is then scraped off at skin level. Because of the burning or drying action of the electric current, there's almost no bleeding.

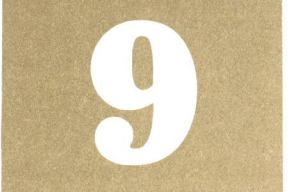

Serious disorders

Carcinoma *is another word for cancer.*

Serious skin disorders like actinic keratoses, scleroderma, discoid lupus erythematosus, and skin cancer are potentially life-threatening. We don't know the causes of some of these diseases, and the treatments haven't yet been perfected. The best defense against these disorders is to pay attention to your skin and its health. Report to your doctor immediately any changes or other symptoms of disease.

Actinic keratoses
These are caused by exposure to the sun and are precancerous lesions. They occur most often in middle-aged or elderly white men with fair skin. When outdoors, people prone to development of actinic keratoses should avoid exposure to the sun. They should wear a sunscreen with maximum sun-filtering ability and wear protective clothing.

Symptoms of actinic keratoses
- The growths are hard and reddish brown.
- They're attached firmly to the skin.
- Because they're the result of sun exposure, they most frequently appear on the face, scalp, ears, hands, and arms.

Treatment for actinic keratoses
Actinic keratoses always require medical treatment because they're precancerous (prone to become malignant). If treated at an early stage, these precancers are highly curable. If neglected, actinic keratoses may spread cancer to the lymph glands and internal organs and may ultimately prove fatal.

1. The chemical 5-Fluoruracil (5FU) may be applied locally by a doctor to kill the potentially malignant cells.

2. Cyrosurgery (liquid nitrogen therapy) utilizes an extremely cold substance that is applied briefly to the keratoses. This causes them to form blisters; the growths drop off in a few days.

Scleroderma
Scleroderma is a mystery disorder that baffles doctors

Tumors *are growths on or in the body that are either benign (harmless) or malignant (cancerous). Almost everyone develops one or more tumors at some point. Fortunately, most of these tumors are benign.*

and scientists. It's a very serious disease with no known cause or cure.

Scleroderma (which means "hardening of the skin") results from a disease of the body's connective tissue, or collagen. The hardening is caused by the disordered collagen replacing the fat that lies under the top skin layers. The skin and underlying tissues reach an almost cementlike hardness. The disease causes hands to become clawlike, immobile, and useless. Fingertip ulcerations and gangrene may occur. Scleroderma affects women far more often than men and usually strikes between the ages of 25 and 55. The disease is progressive, incurable, and unpredictable in its pattern. Periodically, attacks worsen and then subside. Very mild cases occasionally cure themselves.

Symptoms of scleroderma

• The skin loses elasticity and becomes hardened, boardlike, resembling armor plate or an armadillo hide.

• A pattern of hard, smooth, yellow- or ivory-colored plaques develops. These plaques are immobile and are attached to underlying tissue.

• Only a few plaques may appear (a localized form of the disease); or they may cover the face, hands, and feet. However, sometimes the scalp, chest, neck, or thighs are involved.

• In the early stages of the disease, the affected areas are reddened or lilac-colored and swollen. As the disease progresses, the skin becomes thicker, smoother, firmer, drier, and ivory-yellow in color. On the face, scleroderma results in stretched, taut skin, masklike and expressionless in appearance. The features are pinched, puckered, or drawn into a line. Opening the mouth, chewing, blinking the eyes, or moving the neck become difficult.

Treatment for scleroderma

1. Daily exercise is an important part of the scleroderma treatment.

2. Regular massage, maintaining and protecting body warmth, and avoiding injury are also advisable.

3. A warm bath should be taken 2 or 3 times a week. Done properly, this is a lengthy procedure, taking approximately 3 hours each time.

• The water should be heated gradually from 95 degrees F. to 101 degrees F. The patient should bathe until the body temperature reaches 100 to 101 degrees F. Afterward, wrapped in heated cotton blankets, the patient should be put to bed until perspiration stops. The last steps are a thorough drying, an alcohol rub, and sleep for 8 to 10 hours.

> ## *Managing scleroderma*
> You can minimize the effects of scleroderma by doing the following:
> • Report to your doctor any abnormal bruising or nonhealing abrasions immediately. They may indicate bleeding problems.
> • Keep regular appointments with your doctor for periodic laboratory testing to monitor the effects of drugs that lessen or prevent an immune response.
> • Wear warm socks and gloves, and avoid exposure to cold to lessen hand and foot debilitation.
> • Minimize ulcerations on your fingers by avoiding burns and cuts and treating any local infections immediately.
> • Use skin-softening lotions, soaps, and bath oils to prevent skin dryness and cracking.
> • Eat small, frequent meals. Drink liquids with meals. Chew foods slowly and carefully to minimize swallowing difficulty.

Skin cancer
Skin cancer is the most common form of cancer; it's encountered more frequently than all other forms of cancer combined. It's also the easiest form of cancer to treat. This is because skin cancer can be easily seen and detected in its early stages and is accessible for treatment. Skin cancer is also easy to watch for signs of spreading or recurrence.

Possible causes of skin cancer
As with all other kinds of cancer, the causes of skin cancer aren't precisely known. However, certain factors are known to contribute to the development of skin cancers.

• Exposure to the sun
The more your skin is exposed to the sun, the greater your chances of developing skin cancer. Thus, skin cancer is more common in rural areas—where people work outdoors—than in urban areas. Skin cancer is also more common in the South and West than in the North and East simply because people in the South and West spend more time outdoors.

People who work outdoors, such as farmers, ranchers, sailors, and professional athletes, are far

Not an indication
The presence or absence of hair in a mole doesn't indicate a melanoma.

Discoid lupus erythematosus
Discoid lupus erythematosus (DLE) is marked by chronic skin eruptions that can lead to scarring and permanent disfigurement. The exact cause of DLE is unknown. An estimated 60 percent of patients with DLE are women in their late twenties or older. This disease is rare in children.

DLE lesions are raised, red, scaling plaques. The raised edges and sunken centers give them a coinlike appearance. Although these lesions can appear anywhere on the body, they usually erupt on the face, scalp, ears, neck, and arms, or any part of the body that's exposed to sunlight. Hair tends to become brittle or may fall out in patches.

People with DLE should avoid prolonged exposure to the sun, fluorescent lighting, or reflected sunlight. They should wear protective clothing, use sunscreening agents, engage in outdoor activities only in the early morning or late afternoon (before 10 A.M. or after 2 P.M.), and report any changes in the lesions to a doctor.

more prone to skin cancer than people who work indoors.

- Exposure to other irritants

The skin isn't only the body's largest organ—it's the most exposed. Factors such as exposure to chemical irritants and carcinogenic substances contribute to the development of skin cancer.

Symptoms of skin cancer

Skin cancer occurs in three forms: basal cell carcinoma, squamous cell carcinoma, and malignant melanoma.

- Basal cell carcinoma

Basal cell carcinoma is the least dangerous of the three forms of skin cancer. It grows slowly and almost never spreads through the bloodstream to other parts of the body. It appears as a waxy-white lump that may become an open sore. If treated in its early stages, it's almost 100 percent curable; if neglected, it may spread to other areas.

- Squamous cell carcinoma

Squamous cell carcinoma occurs most often in fair-skinned white males over age 60. It's serious because it may grow and spread to the lymph glands and then to other organs.

- Malignant melanoma

Malignant melanoma is one of the most dangerous types of cancer. It's discussed further beginning on page 91.

Treatment for cell carcinomas

Early diagnosis and treatment are essential to the cure of skin cancer. Treatment of a particular skin cancer will depend on its type, location, size, degree to which it has invaded underlying tissue, and whether or not it has spread to other parts of the body (metastasis). The age and health of the patient are also important.

Effective treatment for skin cancer requires removal of the affected skin area.

1. If cancer is suspected, your doctor will perform a biopsy to determine cell type and structure.

2. Treatment may consist of surgery, with or without skin grafting.

3. Curettage (scraping) with electrodesiccation (burning tissue with an electric spark) gives good cosmetic results.

Consult your doctor

Consult your doctor if any "mole," "wart," "pimple," "cold sore," or growth of any kind changes in color, texture, or size or doesn't heal within a month. Also consult your doctor if any new growth suddenly appears on your skin.

Skin cancers usually grow larger. They almost never itch or cause pain, and they don't heal without treatment.

4. Radiation can also be used, either in conjunction with surgery or as the only treatment; X-ray treatment can improve the cure rate. When used alone, radiation does not open the skin surface and does not leave scars. It's also used for elderly or infirm people.

5. To prevent the development of other skin cancers, the patient must avoid exposing the skin to further sun damage.

Melanoma

Melanoma is the most deadly form of skin cancer and one of the most dangerous forms of cancer. This is because it rapidly spreads through the bloodstream and lymph glands to other organs, particularly the brain, lungs, and liver as well as the bones, attacking all the tissue it touches.

Possible causes of melanoma

The cause of melanoma isn't known, but certain factors seem to be related to its occurrence.

• People with light skin, hair, and eye color are more prone to develop melanomas. These people also sunburn more easily, and sun exposure is known to be a contributing factor to skin cancers of all types.

• Melanoma occurs most frequently in geographical areas that are warmer—and sunnier.

Melanoma

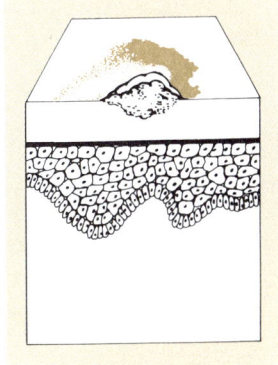

• Black people rarely develop melanomas. However, when they do, the growth usually appears on areas of the skin that have less melanin pigment protection, such as the palms of the hands and the soles of the feet.

• It's more common in women than men and is rare in children.

Symptoms of melanoma

• You should be suspicious if you observe changes in the shape, size, color, or borderline of a mole or if you develop a new mole after age 40. Common sites are the head and neck in men, legs in women, and the backs of people who expose themselves to excessive sunlight.

• Unlike common, harmless moles, melanomas are asymmetrical (they don't have two matched "halves"); their borders are ragged in design (rather than being smooth); and their color tends to be a mixture of shades (rather than only one color).

• A mole that begins to bleed or becomes an open sore may also indicate a melanoma.

Treatment for melanoma

1. If you discover any suspicious mole or growth, consult your doctor. He or she will probably recommend a biopsy or immediate removal of the mole or growth. If a large amount of tissue surrounding a melanoma is removed, skin grafting may be necessary.

2. If the melanoma is detected early enough and surgically removed, 50 percent of cases can be cured.

3. The cure will depend not only on removal of the growth but also on control of the spread of the cancer to underlying skin layers, the lymph system, and other parts of the body.

4. Large tumors may require follow-up chemotherapy. If the disease has spread, radiation treatment will be necessary.

Coping with possible skin cancer

Skin cancers are curable if you find them early and report them to your doctor. Follow these guidelines:

• Examine all your skin surfaces frequently. For difficult to see areas, use a mirror—or two, where necessary. To check your scalp, make regular parts close together or use a hair dryer set on cool, to expose scalp surfaces.

• Check for moles. Look for changes in shape, size, or color. Normal moles have even edges and unchanging color.

• Note all pimples, cold sores, warts, or growths. Check especially for changes in color, texture, or size.

• Check all sores, from their first development to their completed healing.

Bring to your doctor's attention any growth, mole, or skin irregularity that changes in size, shape, color, or sensitivity; any mole or growth that bleeds without being irritated or cut; and any sore that doesn't heal completely in a normal amount of time—a month at the latest.

Index

A
Aberel, 34
Abrasion (for hair removal), 17
Abrasions, 29
Accutane, 34
Acetinic keratoses, 87
Acne, 15, 32-35
 collagen implants, 9
 prevention, 35
 treatment, 33-35
Acylovar, 56
Adenosine phosphate, 56
Alkali in soap, 12
Allergic reactions, 14, 41-51. *See also* Contact dermatitis
 hives, 49, 51
 insect sting–emergency kit, 51
 job-related allergens, 47
 skin tests for, 46
 to chemicals, 43
 to clothing, 42
 to cosmetics, 43
 to household products, 42
 to houseplants, 42
 to jewelry, 42
 to plants and trees, 43-45
 to skin products, 43
 treatment, 46
Aloe ointment for burns, 26
Antigen, 7
Antihistamines to relieve itching, 40
Astringents, 15, 34
Athlete's foot, 70-71

B
Baking soda compress, 37
Bath oils, 13
Bath vs. shower, 13
Beauty marks. *See* Moles
Bites, insect. *See* Insect bites and stings
Blacks
 melanomas in, 91
 sun considerations, 38
Blisters
 around mouth or lips, 52
 eczema, 68
 impetigo, 65
 in mouth, 73
 shingles, 55
Burns, 25-28
 chemical, 28
 first aid for, 26, 27, 28
 first-degree, 26
 internal damage from, 25
 pain patterns of, 25
 second-degree, 26
 skin grafts for, 27-28
Burow's solution, mixing, 37

C
Cancer, skin, 89-92
 causes, 89-90, 91
 early warning signs, 85
 sun exposure and, 37, 87, 89, 91
Canker sores, 71-73
Carcinoma. *See* Cancer, skin
Chemical burns, 28
Chemosurgery, 9
Chicken pox, 53-54
Chlorpromazine, 40
Cleansing cream, 14
Cleansing oil, 14-15
Cold sores, 39, 52-53, 72
Collagen implants, 9

Comedone extractor, caution, 35
Compresses, soothing, 37
Contact dermatitis, 13, 41-47
Cortisone
 and keloids, 10
 and stretch marks, 9
Cosmetics. *See* Allergic reactions
Crabs. *See* Lice
Cryosurgery, 87
Curettage, 90
Curette surgery, 85, 86
Cuts, 29-31

D
Dandruff, 22
Democycline, 40
Depilatories
 chemical, 18
 wax, 19
Dermabrasion, 9
Diaper rash, 65, 66-67
Diet, 22-24
 acne and, 23, 33, 34
 nutritional deficiencies, 72
 RDAs, 23
 weight changes, effects on skin, 24, 82
Discoid lupus erythematosus (DLE), 90
Doxycycline, 40
Drugs
 as allergens, 51
 causing acne, 32
 sun poisoning risk, 39
Dry skin, 13, 14, 15, 16, 83-84
Duofilm, 63

E
Eczema, 68-69
Electrodesiccation, 90

Electrolysis, 19
Electrosurgery, 85, 86
Emergency kit for insect stings, 51
Epinephrine, 51
EpiPen, 51
Eurax, 80
Eyelifts, 83

F
Face care guidelines, 12, 14-16
Facelifts, 83
Facial exercises, caution, 82
Facials
  masks, 15-16
  scrubs, 15
  steam treatment, 16
  toners, 15
Fever blisters, *See* Cold sores
Fibrel, 9
First aid
  burns, 26, 27, 28
  shock (state of), 27
Foot problems, 70-71
Foot soaks, 70
Frostbite, 28-29
Fungal infections, 70-71

G
Genital herpes. *See* Herpes, genital
Genital sores, 57, 75
Grafts, skin, 27-28

H
Hair care, 20-22
Hair removal, 17-19
Hardening skin. *See* Scleroderma
Healing process, 30-31
Heat rash. *See* Prickly heat
Herbal-steam treatment, 16

Herpes, genital, 57-61
  blindness, risk of, 60
  cancer risk, 60
  "HELP" address, 59
  lesion-healing aids, 60
  pregnancy and, 59
  prevention, 61
  symptoms, 58
  treatment, 60-61
  vaccine development, 61
Herpes simplex, 39, 52, 53, 57. *See also* Cold sores
Herpes transmission, 57, 58, 61
Herpes zoster. *See* Shingles
Hives, 49, 51

I
Impetigo, 64-66
Infants
  skin irritants, 67
  skin protectants, 65
Inflammatory dermatitis, 39
Insect bites and stings, 47-51
Insect repellents, 42
  emergency kit, 51
  removing stinger, 50
  treatment, 49-50
Interferon, 63
Itching. *See also* Contact dermatitis and under specific causes
  antihistamines for, 40
  ice to relieve, 49

K
Keratoses, 85-86
Kwell, 78, 80

L
Lice, 76-78
Lupidon, 61
Lupus, 39
Lupus erythematosus, 90
Lye burns, 28
Lysine, 60

M
Masks, facial, 15-16
Melanin, 36-37, 39
Melanomas, 91-92

Men's face care, 16-17
Metastasis, 90
Moisturizers, 15
Moles, 62, 84-85, 90, 91-92
Mouth sores. *See also* Cold sores; Canker sores
  canker sores vs. cold sores, 72

N
Nitric acid burns, 28
Nutritional deficiencies, 24, 72

O
Oil treatment for hair, 21
Oily skin, 15, 16

P
Paint remover burns, 28
Pantothenic acid (for burns), 26
Plucking (hair removal), 17-18
Pock marks, 9
Poison ivy, 44-45
Poison oak, 44-45
Poison sumac, 44-45
Pores, enlarged, 80-81
Prickly heat, 66, 67-68
Psoriasis, 73-76
  symptoms, 74-75
  treatment, 75-76

R
Rash
  lice-caused, 78
  shingles, 55
RDAs (Recommended Dietary Allowances), 23
Retin-A, 34

S
Scabies, 78-80
Scabs from shingles, 55
Scales, psoriasis, 74
Scalp care, 20-22
Scalp massage, 21
Scars, 8-9, 34, 57

Scleroderma, 87-89
Scrapes, 29
Scrubs, facial, 15
Seborrheic keratoses, 85-86
Self-examination for melanomas, 91
Shampooing, 20, 22
Shaving, 18
Shingles, 53-57
    symptoms, 55-56
    treatment, 56-57
Shock (state of)
    first aid, 27
    signs of, 25
Shower vs. bath, 13
Skin cancer. See Cancer, skin
Skin grafts, 27-28
Skin growths, changes in, 91. See also Keratoses; Moles; Warts
Skin hardening. See Scleroderma
Skin structure and functions, 4-8
Skin tests for allergens, 46
Skin toners, 15
Skin type, determining, 14
Smoking, effects on skin, 83
Soap, effects of, 11-13
Sores, genital, 57, 75
Steam-treatment (facial), 16
Stretch marks, 9-10
Sun Protection Factors (SPFs), 38
Sun, effects of, 14, 82, 87, 91
    sunburn, 36-39
    sun poisoning, 39-40
Sunscreen tips, 37, 39

T
Tanning salons, caution, 39
Tetanus immunization, 29, 31
Tetracycline, 39, 40
Topical medications, 7
Tretinoin, 34
Tumors, 88. See also Cancer, skin
Turpentine burns, 28
Tweezing, 17-18

U
Ultraviolet, 39
    for acne, 35
    for eczema, 69
    negative effects, 37

V
Virus-related disorders, 52-63
Vitamins, 24
    acne alleviation, 34
    burn ointment, 26
    causing sun sensitivity, 40
    deficiencies, 24
    scar preventative, 34, 57

W
Warts, 61-63
Washing
    excessive, 11, 83
    techniques, 11-13
Weight changes, effects on skin, 24, 82
Wrinkles, 81-83

Z
Zovirax, 56, 60-61